Three Ingredient Cookbook

LOW-FAT

A Collection of Favorite Recipes
Compiled By

RUTHIE WORNALL

502-95

A Word of Thanks . . .

> *"A recipe not shared with others
> will soon be forgotten."*

I wish to express my sincere appreciation and thanks to all those individuals who donated recipes or in any other way contributed to the publication of this cookbook.

Special thanks to the following people for helping me kitchen test and taste these recipes: Jane Wiss, Carolyn Warren, Tessa McKee, Lois Davis, John Wornall, Jim Wornall, and Velora Holt.

Additional copies of this cookbook can be purchased by sending **$5.95** per copy, plus **$1.05** postage to:

Ruthie Wornall
Wornall Publishing Co.
9800 W. 104th Street
Overland Park, Kansas 66212
(913) 888-1530

ISBN 0-9624467-7-7

printed by
CLASSIC AMERICAN FUNDRAISERS
11184 Antioch, Suite 415
Overland Park, KS 66210

SECOND PRINTING
November 1995

<u>**6,462 books now in print!**</u>

Three Ingredient Cookbook
Low-Fat
by
Ruthie Wornall

When my doctor put me on a low-fat diet, I thought of the expression, "When life gives you lemons, make lemonade." So I decided to write this **Low-Fat 3 Ingredient Cookbook**. The low-fat diet was a "lemon"; this cookbook is the "lemonade."

I wrote this book in the hope that it would help both you and me realize the seriousness of eating too much fat. There are a couple of important points that I want to make.

#1. We're fat because we eat fat! It is mainly the fat calories that count, not the carbohydrate and protein calories. And it is the combination of low-fat diet and exercise that helps us lose weight.

The total amount of fat we eat should be less than 30% of our daily diet. For example, a 2,000 calorie diet which is 30% fat has 66 fat grams. No more than 10% should come from saturated fats. There are 9 calories in 1 gram of fat. If you want to know what percentage of food comes from fat, you simply multiply the fat gram content in each food by 9. If you want to know how much fat you are eating, count fat grams.

Can you believe there are 14 grams of fat in each tablespoon of oil? There are 13.9 grams of fat in a 3 ounce hamburger pattie and 22 grams of fat in a small piece of cheesecake!

#2. Fat increases your risk of heart attacks, strokes, cancer, and obesity. To put it bluntly, too much fat can kill you!

Therefore, everyone, including children, should eat low-fat foods.

The **Low-Fat 3 Ingredient Cookbook** will help you to choose foods low in fat. There are 175 low-fat recipes in all categories in this book, and the number of fat grams is listed below each recipe. Entire dinners can be prepared using this cookbook.

Each recipe is fast, easy, tasty, and economical. It does not take a rocket scientist to prepare these simple recipes!

Listed below is a low-fat menu:

Arlene Matthews's Grilled Lemon Chicken • *Brown Rice*
Martha Breckenridge's Fruit Salad • *Ethel Jones's Broccoli Parmesan*
Myrtle Hull's Applesauce Angel Food Cake • *Lemonade*

Happy low-fat cooking!

Ruthie Wornall

Fat

Fat is the greatest dietary culprit in raising cholesterol and triglyceride levels.

Fats are described as saturated and unsaturated. Saturated fats are found in meat, dairy products, and tropical oils. Unsaturated fats are divided into 2 kinds: monounsaturated and polyunsaturated. These fats are found in vegetable, fish, and nut oils.

Polyunsaturated fats include corn oil, sunflower oil, and safflower oil.

Monounsaturated fats are olive oil, canola oil, and peanut oil. These are the best oils for you. Saturated fats are the worst.

When we eat fat, our bodies store about 97% of it for us.

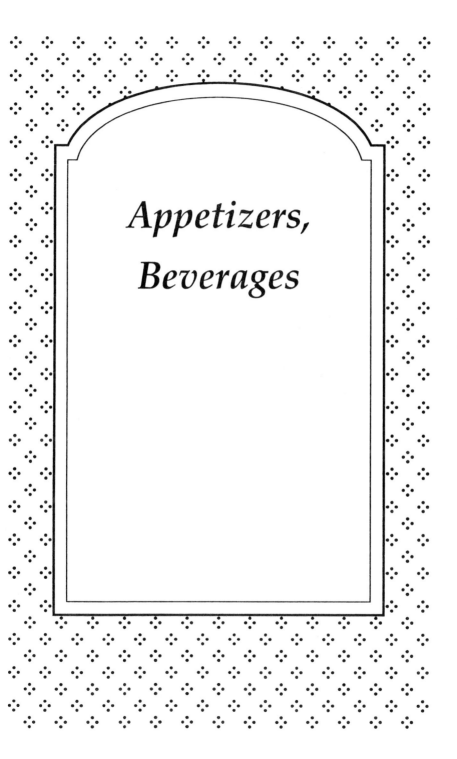

Appetizers, Beverages

A ppetizers are no longer just the special, little morsels served at elegant cocktail parties. They are the snacks and fun food served anytime — mid-afternoon with cold beverages, a snack late at night, as an extra bite that curbs a hungry appetite, or even as the meal itself.

Beverages are important — they cool us, warm us, refresh us, and provide comfort. They are for sharing with friends, sharing with good food, or sharing with just yourself.

HOW TO

The best coffee is made with a clean pot, fresh water, and the right amount of fresh coffee. Begin with 2 tablespoons of coffee for each cup of coffee, then adjust to personal preference. Do not let coffee boil.

Perfect tea is made with freshly boiling water, poured over loose tea or tea bags. Let steep about 5 minutes, and remove tea.

TIMELY IDEAS

Many snacks can be prepared ahead and frozen. Meat and bread combinations freeze especially well. Simply heat and serve. Prepare fresh vegetables the day ahead, but do not freeze. Prepare snacks with eggs, mayonnaise or seafood the day of the party and refrigerate.

Coffee and hot tea should be freshly prepared. Prepare punch or other juice drinks ahead and add the carbonated soda just before serving.

YOUR CREATIVITY

Keep drinks more flavorful, plus make them fun by making your own ice cubes out of juice, tea or another beverage. Add cherries or pineapple cubes for extra color.

TIPS

Keep hot dips or appetizers HOT and cold ones COLD — even during long receptions or parties. They taste better, but the creamy bases lend themselves to bacteria growth so it is essential that the proper temperature is maintained. Prepare small batches and set out only what can be eaten fairly quickly. Have fresh bowls of dip stored in the refrigerator ready to serve. Keep hot snacks in a slow cooker, on a warming tray, or in a fondue pot and replenish them frequently.

Remember plates, forks, and napkins make eating easier. Also, it is almost impossible to have too many glasses or too much ice.

HOW MUCH?

Plan the quantity of appetizers by the meal to follow. If a rich menu is to be served, plan only a serving or two per guest. If the entire menu is appetizers, and guests are to serve themselves, be sure to have plenty of several different varieties.

A standard cup of coffee (used to determine the size of the coffee maker) is about 5 ounces. Coffee mugs hold more, so plan the number of servings needed by the size of the cup, number of guests, and time of day. One pound of coffee makes 40-50 cups.

YOUR HEALTH

Appetizers, snacks and some beverages are known for being high in calories and low in nutrition. Select carefully and you can still enjoy these treats. Select vegetables, fruit, lean meat and low-fat dairy products. These choices are foods that are often low in sodium, low in cholesterol, and high in fiber.

Beverages made of fruit juice, tomato juice, and skim milk are wonderful nutrition sources and can be made into fun, special beverages. Milk punches and shakes provide calcium, protein, and Vitamins A & D.

Any snack or beverage should be counted as part of your total daily food intake. They will supply nutrition plus calories so don't ignore them.

APPETIZERS, BEVERAGES

JANAI'S BEAN AND CHEESE DIP

1 (16 oz.) can non-fat refried   Low-fat Tortilla Chips
  beans
⅓ c. non-fat Cheddar cheese,
  shredded

Spoon beans into a microwave-safe dish and microwave for 2 minutes. Turn dish. Sprinkle cheese over top and microwave until cheese melts, about 1 minute. Serve with Low-fat Tortilla Chips (recipe follows). Yield: 2 cups.

Note: Janai said she often tops this dip with thick and chunky salsa. The bean and cheese dip is fat free. Tortilla chips have 2.7 grams of fat for 20 chips.

JOHN WORNALL'S TORTILLA CHIPS AND DIP

1 pkg. corn tortillas   1 (16 oz.) jar thick and chunky
¼ tsp. cumin seasoning   salsa

Cut a stack of 10 tortillas into 8 wedges each. Spread these "pie-shaped" wedges on a baking sheet that has been sprayed with a non-stick cooking spray. Sprinkle lightly with cumin. Bake at 375°F. for 5 minutes. Turn and bake 5 minutes longer or until chips are crisp. Watch carefully that they do not burn. Cool. Yield: 80 chips or about 4 servings. Serve with salsa.

Twenty chips contain 2.7 fat grams.

EL RANCHO SALSA

1 c. nonfat plain yogurt   3 Tbsp. lite Ranch dressing mix
½ to ¾ c. thick and chunky salsa

Combine all ingredients in a bowl and mix well. Yield: 1½ cups. No fat grams!

Note: This dip is good with homemade low-fat tortilla chips. Great on tacos, too!

TERIYAKI STEAK TIDBITS

1½ lb. flank steak   2 (5 oz.) cans water chestnuts,
⅓ c. bottled teriyaki sauce   drained

Cut flank steak in half lengthwise, then cut in thin diagonal slices across grain. Place meat in bowl. Pour teriyaki sauce over meat and stir

gently to mix. Marinate for 2 hours in the refrigerator. Cut chestnuts into thirds. Roll steak slice around water chestnuts and secure with wooden picks. Broil 3 inches from fire for about 3 minutes. Serve warm. Yield: 50.
Contains about 1 fat gram each.

SHARON HAERTLING'S PARMESAN SQUARES

8 slices white bread, crusts removed

½ c. fat free mayonnaise
½ c. fat free Parmesan cheese

Trim crusts from bread and cut into 4 squares. Mix together mayonnaise and cheese, then spread on bread squares. Place bread on a cookie sheet and bake at 375°F. until bubbly and golden brown.
Optional: Add onion on top of bread before baking.
These squares are less than ½ fat gram each.
Serve as appetizer or with soup or salad.

ARTICHOKE DIP

1 (17 oz.) can artichoke hearts, drained
1 c. fat free mayonnaise

1 env. fat free Italian salad dressing mix

Place artichokes in a blender container and chop, then stir in mayonnaise and Italian dressing mix and blend until creamy.
Serve with fresh vegetables, pretzels, Melba toast or Sharon's Parmesan Squares in the preceding recipe. Yield: 1⅓ cups. Fat free!
Variation: I mixed this dip with tuna and made a tasty sandwich.

CLAM DIP

8 oz. low-fat 1% cottage cheese
1 small can minced clams, drained

Dash of Worcestershire sauce

Place the 3 ingredients in a blender and blend until well-mixed. Yield: 1¼ cups.
Good with lowfat baked Doritos or lowfat potato chips.
Three ounces clams equal 2.5 fat grams. One-half cup 1% cottage cheese equals 1.2 grams of fat.

POTATO CHIPS

4 baking potatoes
Salt or seasoned salt

Paprika

Preheat oven to 300°F. Scrub potatoes and slice as thin as you wish. Place a wire rack in a baking pan and spray with nonstick cooking spray.

Place potato slices in a single layer on the wire rack. Season with salt and paprika. Bake for 50 minutes or until potato chips are crisp and brown. Serves 4.

One potato equals 0.2 grams of fat (negligible fat grams).

LOIS ROHM'S BAGEL APPETIZERS

4 bagels
1 (3 oz.) pkg. nonfat cream
cheese, softened

Stuffed green olives, sliced

Slice bagels crosswise into 4 slices. Brush cut surface of bagel with water. Place on a cookie sheet and bake at 325°F. until crisp and golden, about 15 minutes. Cool.

Spread each slice with softened cream cheese. Sprinkle with sliced green olives. Yield: 16 slices.

One bagel (4 slices) equals 1.4 fat grams. One ounce green olives equals 3.6 fat grams.

Note: The bagel slices can be served without heating for a faster appetizer.

FRUIT ANTIPASTO

Cantaloupe or honeydew melon
slices
Seedless green grapes

Whole strawberries (or apple
wedges)

Cut melon slices in halves crosswise. Arrange melon with small clumps of grapes and strawberries (or apple wedges) on a platter. No fat! Serve with the following fruit dip recipe.

FRUIT DIP

1 (8 oz.) sour cream (lowfat)
1 (7 oz.) jar marshmallow creme

4 Tbsp. strawberry jelly or jam

Mix the 3 ingredients together in a bowl. Cover and refrigerate. Serve with fresh fruit. Yield: About 2 cups.

Contains 1.3 fat grams per tablespoon.

Note: Try non-fat sour cream for a fat free dip.

HORSERADISH DIP

1 (8 oz.) ctn. plain lowfat yogurt
1 Tbsp. low-fat mayonnaise

2 tsp. prepared horseradish

Combine the 3 ingredients in a bowl and mix until well blended. Serve as a dip for fresh vegetables or pretzels. Yield: 1 cup.

Contains 1 fat gram per ounce.
Note: This is a good accompaniment to roast beef.

DOROTHY TOWNSEND'S TURKEY KABOBS

1 lb. unsliced cooked turkey
  breast

32 seedless green grapes
1 c. lowfat creamy dressing

Cut turkey into 1 inch cubes. Arrange a cube of turkey and a green grape on frilled party picks. Arrange around a bowl of salad dressing for dipping. Yield: 32 kabobs.
Contains 1 gram of fat per kabob.

DOROTHY TOWNSEND'S VEGETABLE DIP

1 (24 oz.) ctn. 1% cottage cheese
8 Tbsp. lowfat sour cream

1 (1 oz.) pkg. dry Ranch dressing
  mix

Combine cottage cheese and sour cream and blend until smooth. Stir in dry Ranch dressing mix and blend.
Serve with fresh vegetables. Serves 8 to 12.
Contains 2 grams of fat per serving.

CUCUMBER TEA SANDWICHES

Whole grain bread, cut in circles
Hellmann's mayonnaise (fat
  free)

Cucumber, sliced thin

Spread bread circles lightly with mayonnaise. Top with a cucumber slice.
Optional: Garnish with a tiny parsley sprig dipped in mayonnaise so that it will stick to the cucumber.
Contains 1 fat gram in 1 slice bread or in about 4 bread circles. No fat in mayonnaise or cucumber.

ARTICHOKE-CAVIAR APPETIZERS

1 (17 oz.) can artichoke bottoms
1 (8 oz.) ctn. lowfat or nonfat sour
  cream

1 small jar black caviar

Spread 1 teaspoon sour cream on each artichoke bottom, then spoon ½ teaspoon of caviar on top of sour cream. Serves 6 to 8.
Contains about 1 fat gram for each appetizer. Less if nonfat sour cream is used.

RASPBERRY SPRITZER

1 (16 oz.) pkg. frozen raspberries,   2 c. club soda, chilled
    thawed
1 (24 oz.) bottle white grape juice,
    chilled

Place raspberries in a blender container; cover and puree. Strain and discard seeds.
Combine raspberry puree and grape juice in a pitcher. When ready to serve, stir in chilled club soda. Yield: 1½ quarts.

Contains negligible fat grams.

JOAN LOWE'S FRUIT PUNCH

1 (46 oz.) can Hi-C Punch, chilled   Apple cider to taste
1 (2 liter) bottle Canada Dry
    cranberry ginger ale

All ingredients should be chilled, then mix in a punch bowl when ready to serve. Serves about 25. Fat free!

APPLE CIDER TEA

1 gal. apple cider   1 (12 oz.) can frozen lemonade
2 sticks cinnamon   concentrate

Combine and bring to a boil. Reduce heat and simmer for 5 minutes. Refrigerate any unused portions. Yield: 1 gallon plus.
Contains negligible fat grams!

FRUIT SLUSH

2 c. chilled orange juice   10 frozen strawberries, sliced
1 banana, chopped

Place in blender container and puree. Serve immediately. Serves 2.
Contains less than 1 fat gram per serving.
Note: When my son prepared this recipe, he used 1 (10 ounce) package strawberries instead of 10 frozen strawberries and the result was delicious. You might wish to try it this way, also.

SUNSHINE FRUIT PUNCH

1 (12 oz.) can frozen orange juice,
 thawed
1 (46 oz.) can pineapple
 grapefruit drink

4 bananas, mashed

Dilute orange juice as directed on the can. Refrigerate the orange juice and the pineapple juice. When ready to serve, combine in a punch bowl. Stir in mashed bananas. Serves 24 (4 ounce servings).
Contains less than ½ gram of fat per serving.

STRAWBERRY-ORANGE PUNCH

2 c. fresh strawberries, sliced
2 (12 oz.) cans frozen orange juice
 concentrate

1 (2 liter) bottle Sprite (or ginger
 ale), chilled

Place sliced strawberries in the bottom of a punch bowl. Dilute orange juice as directed on the can, then pour over berries. Add Sprite or ginger ale; stir and serve. Serves about 25.
Optional: A frozen punch ring containing strawberries is a lovely addition to this punch.
Contains negligible fat grams per serving.

CRAN-GRAPE PUNCH

2 qt. cranberry-grape juice,
 chilled
1 (6 oz.) can pink lemonade
 concentrate

1 (32 oz.) bottle sparkling water,
 chilled

Mix the cran-grape juice with the pink lemonade in a punch bowl. When ready to serve, stir in the sparkling water. Serves 20 to 25.
Contains no fat per serving.
Note: The sparkling water I used was "Country Raspberry Clearly Canadian sparkling water," and I thought the punch was delicious.

RED SATIN PUNCH

1 pt. cranberry juice, chilled
1 qt. apple juice, chilled

5 to 6 (10 oz.) cans 7-Up, chilled

At serving time, combine the 2 juices in a punch bowl. Slowly pour 7-Up into mixture. Serves about 25.
Contains no fat grams per serving.

HOT MULLED PINEAPPLE JUICE

1 (46 oz.) can unsweetened   1 (2 inch) piece cinnamon stick
   pineapple juice   Ground cloves to taste

     Combine all ingredients in a saucepan and bring to a boil. Reduce heat and simmer, covered, for 20 minutes. Remove from heat. Discard cinnamon stick. Pour into mugs. Serves 8.
     Contains no fat grams per serving.

FRESHLY SQUEEZED LEMONADE

½ c. lemon juice (freshly   ½ c. sugar (or to taste)
   squeezed)   4 c. cold water

     Mix lemon juice and sugar until sugar dissolves. Stir in cold water and mix well. Refrigerate until serving time. Serves 4. Fat free!

KIDS' PARTY PUNCH

1 small pkg. cherry Kool-Aid,   1 qt. ginger ale, chilled
   prepared
1 (6 oz.) can frozen orange juice
   concentrate

     Mix Kool-Aid as package directs. Stir in orange juice concentrate. (Do not dilute orange juice.)
     When ready to serve, add chilled ginger ale and mix well. Serves 10 to 12. No fat!

HOT COCOA

2 c. skim milk   2 to 3 Tbsp. sugar (or to taste)
1½ Tbsp. cocoa powder

     Combine the 3 ingredients in a saucepan and heat on medium, stirring often, until blended and hot. Yield: 2 cups.
     Contains 1 fat gram per serving.

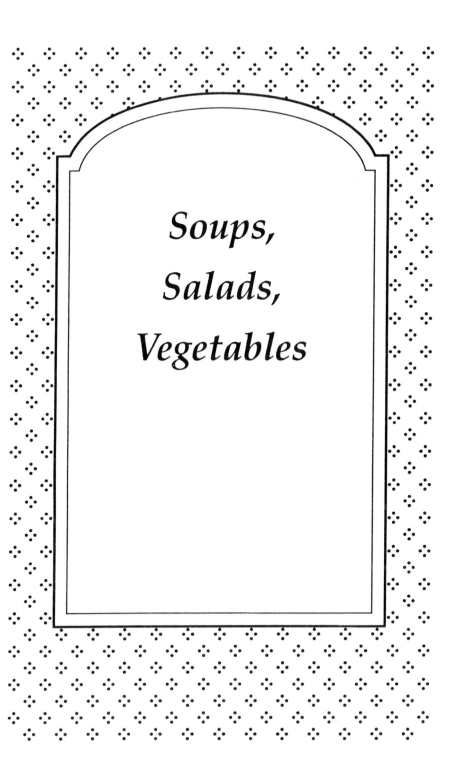

Soups,
Salads,
Vegetables

The crisp crunch of the salads. The tenderness of freshly steamed vegetables. The heartiness and warmth of some soups, while others offer light refreshment. Enjoy these year-round favorites.

HOW TO

Iceburg lettuce can be cut with a knife; all other lettuce should be torn.

For maximum flavor, nutrition, color and texture, cook vegetables only until crisp-tender. Use very little water, keep the pan covered and do not overcook.

TIMELY IDEAS

Soup is best made the day before serving, and refrigerated overnight. The flavors will blend and the fat will solidify on the top so it is easily removed.

Fresh vegetables and lettuce salads are best prepared just before serving. Some salads, like frozen fruit salad, marinated salads, pasta or potato salad and gelatins are best made the day before and refrigerated.

Stir-frying is a quick way to cook vegetables. Heat a small amount of oil in a skillet and add sliced vegetables. Cook over high heat, stirring quickly, just until crisp-tender.

YOUR CREATIVITY

Soups let your creativity shine and are fun and tasty. Start with either your own stock or a commercially prepared soup, then add your favorite ingredients, use up a few leftovers or try your own seasonings.

Vegetables need not be plain. Combine several types to make your own blend. Or add a flavor extra like mushrooms, mint leaves, a squeeze of lemon, any herb, or sunflower seeds.

TIPS

When making soup, tie the whole herbs and spices in cheesecloth. When ready to serve, the "bouquet garni" is easily removed.

If a soup or sauce tastes too salty, add a sliced potato and allow to simmer. Discard potato before serving.

To unmold gelatin, dip it quickly in warm water, then loosen the top edge with a knife. Invert on lettuce-lined plate and shake gently.

Tomatoes are easily peeled when held in boiling water for 30-60 seconds. Plunge in ice water and peel.

HOW MUCH?

For soup, serve ¾ to 1 cup as an appetizer, or 1¼ to 1¾ cups as a main dish.

An average head of iceburg lettuce gives about 10 cups of torn pieces.

A serving of vegetables is ½ cup or about ¼-⅓ pound.

YOUR HEALTH

Salads are almost always the best food choice when counting calories. The exception is when you ladle on the dressing and the extras. In fact, if you use 2 or 3 "ladles" of dressing from the salad bar, you have added 4-6 tablespoons (or ¼ to ⅓ cup) of dressing. If you then add croutons, bacon pieces and cheese, your healthy, low calorie dish is now high in calories and fat. Instead, select fresh greens and vegetables, and add low-calorie dressings, lemon juice, or herb flavored vinegars.

Vegetables are naturally low in sodium. If you must sprinkle something, try an herb instead of salt.

Vegetables and salads are excellent sources of fiber. For added fiber and nutrition, eat them raw and do not peel.

Vegetables are good sources of many vitamins and minerals and some should be eaten daily. Some nutrients are surprising. For example, dark green leafy vegetables, broccoli and cauliflower are good sources of calcium. Tomatoes, broccoli and potatoes (with peel left on) are high in Vitamin C.

SOUPS, SALADS, VEGETABLES

PAT'S CHILLED STRAWBERRY SOUP

2 (10 oz.) pkg. strawberries in
  syrup
½ c. cranberries

1 (8 oz.) ctn. nonfat strawberry
  yogurt

Combine in blender container and blend until smooth. Refrigerate 1 to 2 hours before serving. Serve chilled. Serves 6 to 8. Great summer soup!

Note: This soup came from Pat Neaves' Little Black Cookbook, and is used here with her permission.

Contains less than ½ gram of fat per serving.

JANE WISS' CHICKEN AND DUMPLINGS

1 (10¾ oz.) can chicken broth
1 (10¾ oz.) can lowfat chicken
  and vegetable soup

3 or 4 flour tortillas, cubed

Combine broth and soup in a medium saucepan and bring to a boil. Drop in tortilla cubes. Reduce heat and simmer until "dumplings" are tender. Tortilla cubes will puff up like dumplings. Serves 4.

Contains 4 fat grams per serving.

VEGETABLE PASTA SOUP

1 or 2 (10¾ oz.) cans lowfat
  tomato soup
1 (15 oz.) can mixed vegetables
  (undrained)

1 c. cooked corkscrew macaroni

Cook macaroni as package directs and drain. Dilute soup.

Combine soup and mixed vegetables. Stir in cooked and drained macaroni and heat thoroughly. Season to taste. Serves 4 to 6.

Contains 1½ fat grams per serving.

Optional: I sometimes add chopped onion to this soup (or onion soup mix).

EASY ONION SOUP

1 lb. onions, sliced thin
3 c. beef broth, defatted

2 tsp. Worcestershire sauce

In a medium saucepan, combine onions and beef broth. Simmer 10 to 15 minutes or until onion is soft and translucent. Stir Worcestershire sauce into soup. Ladle into bowls. Serves 4 to 6.

Optional: Sprinkle lowfat cheese over each serving.

Contains no fat grams per serving.

GRACE HEINMAN'S BROCCOLI-CHEESE SOUP

1 (10¾ oz.) can low-fat cream of   4 Tbsp. nonfat Cheddar cheese,
  chicken soup   shredded
1 (10 oz.) pkg. frozen chopped
  broccoli

Cook broccoli as package directs. Stir in soup and mix well. Heat thoroughly. Add shredded cheese and stir until melted. Serves 4.

Contains about 1½ fat grams per serving.

Note: This recipe is in memory of a wonderful woman. Grace gave me this recipe a week or two before she went to heaven.

BLACK BEAN SOUP

2 (15 oz.) cans black beans   1 tsp. lime juice
1 small onion, chopped

Spray a skillet with a nonstick cooking spray and saute the chopped onions until they are soft. Add more cooking spray if needed. Stir in beans and bring to a boil. Reduce heat. Mash about half of the mixture with a fork to add body to the soup. Simmer for 15 minutes. Stir in lime juice just before serving. Serves 4.

Contains 1 fat gram per serving.

MINTED GREEN PEA SOUP

2 (10¾ oz.) cans low-fat   1 (8 oz.) can green peas
  condensed green pea soup   1 Tbsp. chopped mint

Dilute 1 can of green pea or split pea soup in a saucepan. Stir in second can of soup, but do not dilute. Add can of undrained green peas and mix well. Heat to boiling point, then reduce heat and simmer for 5 minutes. Pour soup into bowls and sprinkle each with chopped mint. Serve hot. Serves 4.

Contains less than 2 fat grams per serving if low-fat soup is used.

TEX-MEX VEGETABLE SOUP

2 (15 oz.) cans pinto beans
1 (15 oz.) can whole kernel corn
2 (14½ oz.) cans stewed tomatoes
  with onions, peppers, and
  garlic

Combine all vegetables with their liquids in a large saucepan and heat to boiling. Reduce heat and simmer about 20 minutes. Serves 6 to 8.
Contains less than ½ fat gram per serving.
Optional: You might prefer to cook dried pinto beans instead of using cans.
For a hotter soup, you might want to substitute 2 cans of Ro-Tel tomatoes and chilies, or you could use a 14½ ounce can diced tomatoes with chili seasonings in the sauce.

CREAM OF ASPARAGUS SOUP

2½ c. chopped asparagus   2 to 3 c. low-fat chicken soup
1 small chopped onion

Steam asparagus and onion. Cool. Puree in blender. Heat chicken soup. Stir in asparagus and onion and heat thoroughly. Serves 4.
Contains 1½ fat grams per serving.

MARY RUTH FERRARO'S OKRA GUMBO

2 c. fresh okra, sliced   1 chopped onion
2 c. fresh tomatoes, chopped

Combine in saucepan and bring to a boil. Reduce heat and simmer for 1 hour. Serves 4.
Contains ½ fat gram per serving.
Optional: Substitute a can of stewed tomatoes for fresh tomatoes.

STRAWBERRY SOUFFLE SALAD

1 (3 oz.) pkg. strawberry Jell-O   1 c. boiling water
  gelatin   1 c. mashed strawberries

Stir until Jell-O is dissolved in the boiling water. Add mashed berries and mix. Refrigerate until mixture begins to thicken, then whip with an eggbeater or electric mixer to a very stiff froth.
Serve in sherbet dishes or in any small bowls. Serves 4.
Contains negligible fat grams.

MARTHA BRECKENRIDGE'S FRUIT SALAD

2 c. seedless grapes (red and green)

2 c. cubed cantaloupe
1 to 2 c. sliced strawberries

Combine, mix, and refrigerate until serving time. Serves 6. Contains about 1 gram of fat per cup.

NANCY McDONALD'S MELON COOLER

2 c. lemon-lime carbonated beverage

1 (3 oz.) pkg. orange gelatin
1½ c. diced cantaloupe melon

Bring 1 cup carbonated beverage to bowl. Add to gelatin and stir until dissolved. Stir in 1 cup chilled carbonated beverage and mix well. Cover and refrigerate until partially thickened. Remove from refrigerator and fold in diced melon. Return to refrigerator until firm. Serves 4.
Contains no fat grams!

PAT'S APPLE SALAD

1 (3 oz.) pkg. black cherry Jell-O
3 or 4 apples, peeled, cored, and grated

½ tsp. cinnamon

Prepare Jell-O as package directs. Chill until partially congealed. Stir in grated apples and cinnamon. Cover and return to refrigerator. Chill until firm. Serves 4.
Contains no fat grams.

RASPBERRY-CRANBERRY SALAD

1 (6 oz.) sugar-free raspberry Jell-O
1 (15 oz.) can whole berry cranberry sauce

1 (15 oz.) can crushed pineapple (do not drain)

Prepare Jell-O by mixing and dissolving it in 2 cups boiling water. Stir in pineapple, cranberries, and their juice. Mix well. Cover and refrigerate until congealed. Serves 8.
Contains no fat grams.

APRICOT SALAD

1 (3 oz.) pkg. apricot Jell-O gelatin

1 c. hot orange juice
1 c. cold buttermilk

Dissolve Jell-O in hot orange juice. Mix well. Blend in buttermilk. Pour into a 1 quart mold or dish of your choice and chill until set. Serves 4.

Note: Buttermilk contains 2.2 grams of fat per cup. One cup of orange juice contains 0.5 fat. Jell-O has no fat. Total: 2.7 fat for 4 servings or about 0.6 gram of fat per serving.

TUNA SALAD FLORENTINE

2 c. torn fresh spinach (into bite-size pieces)
2 plum tomatoes, sliced

1 small (3¾ oz.) can water-packed tuna, drained and flaked

Combine spinach, tomatoes, and tuna in a bowl and toss lightly. Serves 2.

Contains 1½ grams of fat per serving.

Note: Serve with nonfat Italian dressing if desired.

JUDY MUELLER'S HONEY-LIME DRESSING

¼ c. fresh lime juice
⅛ c. honey

¼ tsp. Dijon mustard

Mix the 3 ingredients together. Cover and refrigerate! Serve chilled over lettuce or fruit salads. Yield: ⅓ cup. Fat free!

Note: Judy serves this dressing over a romaine and honeydew melon salad.

PEACH MEDLEY

1 (8 oz.) can pineapple chunks and juice
1 (15 oz.) can pear halves, partially drained

1 (15 oz.) can peach halves, partially drained

Combine the 3 canned fruits, using only a little juice from the pears and peaches. Serves 4 to 6.

Optional: Sprinkle with cinnamon.

LOIS ROHM'S BOW TIE PASTA SALAD

1 (16 oz.) pkg. bow tie pasta
1 (16 oz.) pkg. frozen broccoli, cauliflower, and carrots

1 c. low-fat Italian or creamy Italian salad dressing

Prepare pasta as package directs and drain. Cook and drain vegetables. Cool.

Combine all ingredients in a bowl and mix well. Refrigerate until well-chilled. Serves 8.

Contains about 1 fat gram per serving.

Optional - Add any of these following ingredients if you wish: Sliced ripe olives, chopped green onions, cubes of cheese, chicken or turkey.

FROZEN FRUIT SALAD

1 (30 oz.) can apricot halves,   3 sliced bananas
  drained   1 (6 oz.) can frozen orange juice

Place all ingredients in a blender and blend until smooth. Place cupcake paper liners in muffin tins and fill with fruit mixture. Leave paper liners of salad in muffin tins. Cover and freeze until firm. Remove salads from tin and store in plastic bags. Seal and keep in freezer. Thaw for 15 minutes before serving. Serves 8.

Contains less than 1 fat gram per serving.

STUFFED GREEN PEPPER SALAD

4 green peppers   1 chopped onion (red)
2 c. cottage cheese (2%)

Cut a slice from the tops of each green pepper. Remove pith and seeds. Combine chopped red onion and lowfat 2% cottage cheese. Stuff peppers. Refrigerate until serving time. Serves 4.

Contains 2 fat grams per serving.

WILMA RICHEY'S CHERRY-RASPBERRY SALAD

1 (3 oz.) pkg. raspberry Jell-O   1 c. boiling water
1 (21 oz.) can cherry pie filling

Dissolve Jell-O as directed on the package in 1 cup boiling water, but do not add cold water. Stir cherries into dissolved Jell-O. Pour into a 4 cup mold or 9x9 inch dish. Refrigerate until firm. Serves 4.

Contains no fat grams!

WALDORF SALAD

1 c. 1% cottage cheese (low-fat)   1 stalk celery, chopped
1 apple, diced (Red Delicious
  apple)

Combine, mix, cover, and refrigerate. Serves 1 or 2.

Contains 1½ fat grams for 1 serving, less than 1 fat gram for 2 servings.

DORIS HANKS' TOMATO-ASPARAGUS SALAD

2 fresh tomatoes   1 head romaine lettuce
1 lb. fresh asparagus spears

    Slice tomatoes. Cook fresh asparagus in boiling water for 5 to 6 minutes or until tender. Drain. Chill asparagus.
    Line 4 salad plates with romaine lettuce leaves. Top with additional lettuce that had been torn in bite-size pieces. Arrange chilled asparagus spears and tomato slices over the lettuce. Serves 4. Fat free!
    Optional: If desired, drizzle with fat-free Italian salad dressing.

HEAVENLY HASH

2 (16 oz.) cans fruit cocktail,   2 bananas, sliced
  drained   1 c. mini marshmallows

    Combine, mix, and chill. Serves 6. Fat free!

TESSA McKEE'S ORANGE SALAD

1 small pkg. sugar-free orange   2 carrots, grated fine
  gelatin   1 c. plain low-fat yogurt

    Prepare gelatin as package directs. Refrigerate until partially thickened. Fold in carrots and yogurt. Cover and refrigerate until firm. Serves 4.
    Contains 1 fat gram per serving.

JESSICA WORNALL'S SOUTHWESTERN BAKED POTATOES

4 baking potatoes   4 Tbsp. nonfat Cheddar cheese,
1 (8 oz.) jar thick and chunky   shredded
  salsa

    Wash potatoes and prick their skins several times. Bake for 1 hour or until tender at 400°F. (Do not wrap potatoes in foil.)
    Split tops of potatoes. Spoon desired amount of salsa into each. Top with shredded Cheddar cheese. Serves 4.
    Contains 1 fat gram per potato.

ETHEL JONES' BROCCOLI PARMESAN

1 (10 oz.) pkg. frozen broccoli,   Butter Buds sprinkles
  thawed   Nonfat Parmesan cheese

    Cook broccoli as package directs. Drain. Sprinkle generously with Butter Buds and Parmesan cheese. Serves 4. Fat free!

VELMA STEWART'S ROASTED POTATOES

5 white Idaho potatoes   Seasoned salt
1 onion, quartered or sliced

Cut potatoes into wedges or in large "Texas-cut" French fries. Slice onions in lengthwise strips.

Spray bottom of 9x13 inch pan with a non-fat cooking spray. Place potatoes and onions in pan and spray vegetables with cooking spray.

Bake at 400°F. for 40 minutes or until tender. Sprinkle with salt. Serves 4 to 5.

Contains 1 fat gram per serving.

HAWAIIAN CARROTS

1 (15 oz.) can sliced carrots,   ⅓ c. crushed pineapple and juice
   drained   ½ c. orange juice

Mix all ingredients in a saucepan and cook over low heat until carrots are thoroughly heated. Serves 4.

Contains about ½ fat gram per serving.

LOIS DAVIS' OVEN BAKED FRENCH FRIES

2 lb. large baking potatoes,   1 tsp. chili powder
   scrubbed   1 Tbsp. olive oil

Cover a large baking sheet with foil and spray with a nonstick cooking spray. Preheat oven to 475°F. Place baking sheet in oven to heat it.

Slice potatoes in strips. Sprinkle with chili powder. Toss in bowl or plastic bag to cover. Sprinkle oil over potatoes and toss again. Arrange potatoes on the hot baking sheet. Spray potatoes with the nonstick cooking spray. Bake 20 minutes at 475°F. Turn potatoes over and bake 15 to 20 minutes longer or until golden brown. Serves 6.

Contains 2½ fat grams per serving.

MEXICAN BLACK-EYED PEAS

1 (15 oz.) can black-eyed peas   2 to 3 Tbsp. thick and chunky
1 Tbsp. dry onion flakes   salsa (or to taste)

Heat together in a saucepan until hot. Serves 4. Fat free!

SHARON HAERTLING'S MARINATED VEGETABLES

1 c. fresh broccoli florets   Fat free Italian dressing
1 c. fresh cauliflower florets

Pour broccoli and cauliflower into a bowl and toss with desired amount of fat-free Italian dressing. Marinate in refrigerator. Serves 4. <u>Fat free!</u>

SHELLY GREEN BEANS

1 (15 oz.) can cut green and shelly   1 small chopped onion
  beans   3 Tbsp. chili sauce

Spray a nonstick skillet with a nonstick cooking spray and saute chopped onions. Stir in beans and chili sauce. Cook over medium heat until much of the liquid from the beans has evaporated. Serves 4. <u>Fat free!</u>

STEAMED CABBAGE

1 medium head cabbage,   2 chicken bouillon cubes
  quartered   ½ c. boiling water

Dissolve the bouillon cubes in ½ cup boiling water. Add the cabbage and bring to a boil again. Cook for 5 minutes or until tender. Serves 4 to 6.
Contains about ½ gram of fat per serving.

BAKED SQUASH

3 small acorn squash   ¼ tsp. cinnamon
2 c. apple cider

Cut squash in halves lengthwise. Remove seeds and rinse with cool water. Pour cider into a baking dish. Sprinkle with cinnamon. Place squash, cut side down, in the dish. Bake at 350°F. for 45 minutes. Turn cut side up and spoon cider into cavity. Bake 10 minutes longer or until tender. Serves 6.
Contains <u>no fat grams!</u>

MARILYN WEAVER'S GREEN BEANS

1 (15 oz.) can green beans   1 Tbsp. dehydrated onion flakes
1 to 1½ tsp. beef instant bouillon
  (granules)

Combine the 3 ingredients in a saucepan and mix well. Bring to a boil. Stir, reduce heat, and simmer for 5 minutes. Serves 4.
Contains less than ½ fat gram per serving.

BERRY SWEET POTATOES

1 (1 lb. 2 oz.) can sweet potatoes, 1 c. miniature marshmallows
  sliced
1 (10 oz.) pkg. cranberry-orange
  relish

Place sliced potatoes in a baking dish that was sprayed with nonstick cooking spray. Spread cranberry relish evenly over potatoes. Bake 30 minutes in 350°F. oven. Sprinkle with marshmallows and broil until lightly browned. Serves 6.
Contains no fat!

ETHEL JONES' STEAMED ASPARAGUS

1 lb. fresh asparagus   Butter Buds sprinkles
Juice of 1 lemon

Wash asparagus. Place on a vegetable steamer rack over boiling water. Cover and steam about 6 minutes or until tender. Sprinkle with lemon juice and Butter Buds. Serves 4. Fat free!

MARY DITSCH'S SCALLOPED TOMATOES

1 (14½ oz.) can stewed tomatoes   1 slice wheat toast, cut into cubes
  with onion   1 tsp. Butter Buds sprinkles

Heat tomatoes in a small microwave-safe dish for about 2 minutes on HIGH. Remove from microwave and stir in toast cubes. Sprinkle Butter Buds over top. Return to microwave and heat for 1 minute longer. Serves 4.
Contains ½ gram of fat per serving.

CANDIED SWEET POTATOES

4 sweet potatoes, peeled and cut   2 to 3 Tbsp. raisins
  into chunks   ½ c. brown sugar

Place potatoes in a pan that was sprayed with a vegetable nonstick cooking spray. Sprinkle raisins over potatoes. Top with a thin layer of brown sugar. Cover and bake at 350°F. until tender. Serves 4 to 6.
Contains no fat!

JUDY MUELLER'S MASHED POTATOES

4 or 5 potatoes, peeled and sliced   Evaporated skim milk
Butter Buds sprinkles

Boil potatoes until tender and drain. Generously sprinkle Butter Buds sprinkles over potatoes and mix well. Cover with a lid and let set for 3 minutes. Mash potatoes with desired amount of evaporated skim milk. Serves 4.

Contains 1 fat gram per serving.

BANANA RICE

1 c. brown rice   Butter Buds sprinkles
1 or 2 sliced bananas

Prepare rice as package directs, except do not use butter. Butter Buds sprinkles may be used.

Stir bananas into cooked rice and bake at 375°F. for 10 to 15 minutes. Serves 4.

Optional: Stir banana slices into hot, cooked rice and serve without baking.

Contains less than 1 gram of fat per serving.

ROBIN O'HARA'S LOWFAT PASTA

1 (12 oz.) pkg. spaghetti (lowfat)   No-fat Parmesan cheese
½ (8 oz.) bottle non-fat Italian
  dressing

Cook spaghetti as package directs. Drain. Toss with dressing until coated. Sprinkle with Parmesan cheese. Serves 6.

Contains about 1 fat gram per serving.

DESIREE'S PASTA MARINARA

1 pkg. pasta (of choice)   Fat free Parmesan cheese
1 (14 oz.) jar low-fat marinara
  sauce

Heat marinara sauce. Cook pasta as package directs. Drain. Pour pasta onto a platter. Top with hot marinara sauce and sprinkle generously with Parmesan cheese. Serves 4.

Contains 1½ fat grams per serving.

Main Dishes

J ust as the name says, the main dish is the center of the meal. Say farewell to boring meals and let your creativity soar as you try new recipes, change meat cuts, taste different fish or seafood varieties, or add new seasonings to poultry.

HOW TO

Roasting means to cook meat uncovered, without added liquid. Roasting or broiling is used to cook tender cuts of meat like rib roasts, steaks, chops, or "broiler/fryer" chickens.

Braising is cooking covered, with liquid. Braising or otherwise cooking with liquid is used for less-tender cuts of meat like chuck, round, flank, brisket or hens.

Fish is categorized as "fat" or "thin." Fat fish includes trout, salmon, or tuna, and is best prepared with dry heat, like baking or broiling. Thin fish includes cod, haddock, halibut, perch, orange roughy, or snapper and is best cooked with moist heat, like steaming or poaching. If cooked with dry heat, thin fish should be basted often.

TIMELY IDEAS

Prepare a larger main dish and freeze part for use another day. It is also easy to use a meat in another entree. For example, try roasted chicken in enchiladas, leftover roast in barbecue sandwiches, ham in an omelet or quiche, or turkey with pasta.

Meat and poultry products freeze well if wrapped tightly. For easier use, freeze them in portions sized for your family or recipe. Chicken can be separated into pieces before freezing, so you may cook the piece or quantity needed.

Make hamburger patties, separate with wax paper and freeze. Then they are easy to cook quickly.

YOUR CREATIVITY

A marinade will not only improve the flavor of meat, but will also tenderize it. Experiment with wine-vinegar, salad dressing or fruit juice. Add seasonings like pepper, or herbs.

TIPS

The oven does not need to be preheated when cooking most meats or main dishes.

A meat thermometer is the best way to check meats or poultry for doneness. Insert it into the center, away from bones. Temperatures should read:

Beef	Rare	140	Pork	170
	Medium	160	Poultry	185
	Well	170		

HOW MUCH?

Beef/Pork	Boneless	3-4 servings per pound
	Bone-in	2-3 servings per pound
	Bony (ribs)	1 serving per pound
Fish fillets		2-3 servings per pound
Poultry	Chicken	2-3 servings per pound
	Turkey	1 serving per pound

YOUR HEALTH

Today's meat is leaner than before. There are over fifteen cuts of beef, pork, lamb and veal under 200 calories per 3-ounce serving.

Meats are rich sources of protein, iron, B-vitamins, zinc and other essential nutrients. To balance your intake of fat and cholesterol, don't eliminate meat. Instead select lean cuts, trim fat, and bake or broil. Avoid frying and/or rich gravy.

Removing the skin from chicken saves about 20 calories per serving.

Cook meat on a rack so the fat will drain off.

Meatless main dishes can be nutritious if foods are carefully combined to provide complete proteins. Combine cereals or grains with beans. Serve beans with nuts.

MAIN DISHES

ARLENE MATHEWS' GRILLED LEMON CHICKEN

4 chicken breast halves, skinned ½ c. lemon juice
  and boned 2 to 3 Tbsp. Worcestershire sauce

Trim chicken of all visible fat. Combine lemon juice and Worcestershire sauce. Place chicken breasts in mixture and refrigerate for 1 hour, turning every 15 minutes. Remove from marinade and grill over hot coals, or broil under broiler for about 6 minutes on each side or until tender. Chicken could also be baked for 1 hour at 325°F. Turn after 30 minutes if desired. Serves 4.

Contains 2 to 3 fat grams per serving. (One fat gram counter book said 2 fat grams and another one said 3 fat grams for 1 chicken breast half.)

OVEN-FRIED CHICKEN

4 chicken breasts, halved, 1 Tbsp. canola oil or olive oil
  skinned, and boned 1 oz. wheat germ (or ⅛ c.)

Trim all visible fat from chicken. Rinse chicken with cool water. Dry with paper towels. Lightly brush each chicken breast with oil. (Try to use less than 1 teaspoon of oil on each piece as oil has 14 grams of fat per tablespoon.) Roll in wheat germ. (Try to use about 2 teaspoons on each piece as wheat germ contains 3 fat grams per ounce.)

Place chicken on a foil-lined pan that was sprayed with a nonstick cooking spray and bake at 400°F. for 30 minutes. Turn chicken and bake 15 to 20 minutes longer or until fork tender. Serves 4.

Contains about 6½ fat grams per serving.

SHARON HAERTLING'S PASTA AND CHICKEN

1 (8 oz.) pkg. rigatoni pasta (or 1 (14 oz.) jar chunky garden-style
  pasta of your choice) pasta sauce
4 chicken breast halves, skinned
  and boned

Use pasta that is <u>not</u> made with egg yolks. Prepare as package directs. Drain.

Trim all visible fat from chicken. Place chicken in a pan that has been sprayed with a non-fat cooking spray. Spray tops of chicken with the cooking spray and bake 30 minutes at 325°F. Turn chicken and bake about 30 minutes more or until tender. Cut chicken in strips.

Heat pasta sauce until hot.

To serve, place pasta on each dinner plate. Top with 1 sliced chicken breast on each. Pour hot pasta sauce over all. Serves 4.

Contains 3 fat grams per serving.

Optional: Sprinkle with non-fat Parmesan cheese.

TWYLIA CHURCH'S HERBED CHICKEN

6 boneless, skinless chicken
breast halves
1 env. Lipton's savory herb with
garlic

1 Tbsp. olive oil

Trim all visible fat, then arrange chicken in a 9x13 inch baking pan that has been sprayed with a nonstick cooking spray.

In a small bowl, combine the savory herb mix with 1 tablespoon olive oil and 2 tablespoons of water and mix well. Brush mixture on chicken and bake, uncovered, for 45 minutes to 1 hour or until tender. Serves 6.

Contains about 4½ fat grams per serving.

CURRIED CHICKEN BREASTS

4 chicken breasts, halved,
skinned, and boned
1 (10¾ oz.) can Healthy Choice
lowfat cream of chicken soup

1 tsp. curry powder

Lightly brown chicken breasts in a skillet sprayed with nonfat cooking spray.

Place in a baking dish also sprayed with nonfat cooking spray. Mix soup and curry together. Pour over chicken breasts. Bake 40 minutes at 350°F. or until tender. Makes 4 servings.

Contains 3 fat grams per serving.

LOIS ROHM'S CHICKEN AND PASTA

1 lb. chicken breasts (skinless and
boneless)
1 (10¾ oz.) lowfat cream of
chicken soup, diluted

1 (16 oz.) pkg. frozen seasoned
pasta and vegetable
combination

Cut chicken into cubes. Spray nonfat, nonstick cooking spray in a skillet and brown chicken cubes, turning often. Stir in soup diluted with ½ cup water. Add pasta and vegetable combo and mix well. Cover with a lid and cook 5 to 10 minutes or until chicken is tender and all ingredients are hot. Serves 4.

Contains 3 fat grams per serving.

GRANOLA BAKED CHICKEN

6 to 8 chicken breasts, halved,   1 c. low-fat granola crumbs,
   skinned, and boned   blended to corn meal
½ c. skim milk   consistency

Dip chicken breasts into milk, then roll in granola, which has been made into crumbs by blending it in a blender. Place chicken in a greased 9x13 inch baking dish and bake at 350°F., uncovered, for about 1 hour. Turn after 30 minutes if you wish. Serves 6 to 8.

Contains about 2½ fat grams per serving.

ONITA COPELAND'S "FRIED" CHICKEN

2 chicken breast halves, skinned   2 tsp. olive oil
   and boned   Mrs. Dash seasoning

Spray a skillet with a nonstick cooking spray. Trim any visible fat from chicken.

Rub ½ teaspoon olive oil on each side of the 2 chicken breasts. Sprinkle with Mrs. Dash seasoning. Saute in skillet until golden brown. Turn over and cook on other side until tender and brown. Add more cooking spray if needed. Serves 2.

Contains 7 grams of fat per serving.

Note: This recipe would have only 2 fat grams per serving if you do not use olive oil. You could substitute a nonfat cooking spray for the olive oil and spray it on both sides of the chicken. There is an olive oil nonfat cooking spray on the market.

BEV WEST'S CRANBERRY SAUCE FOR CHICKEN

1 (16 oz.) can whole berry   1 (8 oz.) bottle lowfat French
   cranberry sauce   dressing
1 pkg. onion soup mix

Cranberry Sauce: Combine the 3 ingredients in a bowl and mix until well-blended. Refrigerate, covered, until ready to use. Yield: 3 cups. Fat free.

To prepare chicken, place 8 boneless, skinless chicken breast halves in an oblong Pyrex glass dish and pour Cranberry Sauce evenly over chicken. Cover and marinate overnight in the refrigerator. The next day, bake at 350°F. for 1 hour or until tender. Serves 8.

Contains 2½ fat grams per serving.

Note: This recipe sounds awful, but tastes delicious! It will surprise you!

CHICKEN DIJON

4 to 6 chicken breasts, boned and   Dijon mustard
    skinned
Finely crumbled seasoned bread
    crumbs

Place chicken breasts in a greased baking dish and bake at 350°F. for 20 minutes. Remove from heat. Generously spread Dijon over chicken on both sides, then coat with bread crumbs and return to baking dish. Bake 1 hour longer at 350°F. or until tender. The mustard gives the chicken a tangy flavor and makes it moist. Don't overcook. Serves 4 to 6.
Contains 2½ fat grams per serving.

DOROTHY TOWNSEND'S APRICOT CORNISH HENS

3 (1 lb.) Cornish hens, skinned   3 Tbsp. apricot jam, melted
⅔ c. apricot nectar

Remove giblets from hens. Rinse hens under cold water and pat dry. Split each hen in half lengthwise, using an electric knife. Place hens in a 9x13 inch baking dish. Pour apricot nectar over them, turning to coat. Cover hens with fork and marinate in the refrigerator for 2 hours, turning occasionally. Remove hens from marinade, but reserve marinade.
Bake, uncovered, in a 9x13 inch baking dish that is sprayed with a non-stick cooking spray at 350°F. for 20 minutes. Baste with marinade. Bake 20 minutes longer and baste with melted apricot jam. Bake 20 minutes more or until tender. Serves 6.
Contains 6 grams of fat per serving.

GRILLED CHICKEN KABOBS

4 boneless, skinless chicken   2 or 3 green peppers, cut in cubes
    breast halves
1 (20 oz.) can pineapple chunks,
    drained

Bake chicken at 350°F. for 30 minutes. Remove from oven and cut into 1 inch cubes. Thread alternately on skewers the chicken, pineapple, and green pepper cubes. Grill until chicken and peppers are fork tender. Yield: 16 kabobs.
Contains ½ gram of fat per kabob.

LOUISE HOLTZINGER'S CHICKEN SANDWICH SPREAD

4 ground baked chicken breast   Green pickle relish to taste
    halves, skinned and boned   Low-fat mayonnaise

Bake chicken at 325°F. for 1 hour. Turn over after 30 minutes. Cool. Grind or chop finely the baked chicken breasts. Stir in desired amount of pickle relish and low-fat mayonnaise. Mix well. Serve as a sandwich spread for toast or use to stuff tomatoes. Serves 4 to 6.

Contains 3 fat grams per serving.

JANE BALLARD'S CAJUN CHICKEN

4 boneless, skinless chicken breast halves

Tabasco sauce
Onion powder

Rinse chicken in cool water and dry. Generously sprinkle Tabasco sauce on each side, then season each side with onion powder.

Spray skillet with a non-stick cooking spray. Place chicken in skillet and brown. Turn and brown other side. Cover and cook slowly until fork tender. Serves 4. Hot and spicy!

Contains 2 fat grams per serving.

GRILLED CATALINA CHICKEN

4 skinless, boneless chicken breast halves

½ c. low-fat Catalina dressing
¼ tsp. black pepper

Trim all visible fat from chicken. Mix Catalina dressing and black pepper together. Pour into an oblong dish. Add chicken and turn to coat. Marinate chicken 4 to 6 hours or overnight.

When ready to grill, prepare coals and grill chicken for 20 minutes over hot grill. Brush chicken with reserved marinade. Serves 4.

Contains 4 grams of fat per serving.

ORANGE STUFFED ROAST TURKEY

1 (12 lb.) turkey, skinned
4 oranges, quartered
½ c. liquid Butter Buds (or non-fat butter-flavored cooking spray)

Wash and dry turkey. Remove giblets and neck.

Prepare Butter Buds as package directs to make ½ cup of liquid Butter Buds. Rub on outside of turkey. (Or, spray generously with a butter-flavored nonfat cooking spray.) Fill cavity with orange quarters.

Place turkey, breast up, on a rack in a roasting pan. Follow directions on turkey, wrapping for roasting, or roast at 325°F. for 3½ to 4 hours or until turkey is tender. Serves 20.

Contains 7 fat grams per 3½ ounce serving.

SAGE ROASTED TURKEY BREAST

1 (3 lb.) turkey breast, skinned   Sage
½ c. liquid Butter Buds

Remove skin from turkey breast. Prepare Butter Buds as package directs, then rub over turkey. Sprinkle with sage.

Roast, breast up, on a rack in a roasting pan at 325°F. for about 1½ hours or according to directions on the wrapper. Protect bird with a tent of foil when it is golden brown. Serves 12.

Contains 3 fat grams per 3½ ounce serving.

TURKEY BREAST STEAKS

4 (3½ oz.) white meat turkey   ½ c. dry bread crumbs
  steaks, skinned   (seasoned)
½ c. nonfat Italian salad dressing

Dip steaks in salad dressing, then roll in seasoned bread crumbs.

Spray skillet with nonstick, nonfat cooking spray and saute on both sides until lightly browned and tender. Serves 4.

Contains 7 grams of fat per serving.

POACHED TURKEY BREAST

2 lb. fresh or frozen turkey breast,   1 tsp. lemon juice
  skinned   Boiling water

Remove skin from turkey. Place in a steamer over boiling water. Sprinkle lemon juice over it. Steam for 30 to 35 minutes or until tender and juices run clear when pricked with a fork. Serves 6 to 8.

Contains about 3 grams of fat per 3 ounce serving.

TURKEY AND CRANBERRY SANDWICH

2 thin smoked turkey slices (98%   2 whole grain bread slices
  fat free)
2 Tbsp. whole berry cranberry
  sauce

Toast bread if you wish. Spread cranberry sauce on bread and top with turkey slices. Cut sandwich in half. Yield: 1 serving.

Contains about 3 fat grams per serving.

Note: You can also buy **fat free** slices of turkey breast, then the sandwich would be 2 fat grams as the 2 bread slices are 1 fat gram each.

BOUILLON ROAST TURKEY

1 (12 oz.) turkey, skinned   3½ c. boiling water
4 chicken bouillon cubes

Remove all visible fat. Place prepared turkey on a rack in a roasting pan so that fat will drain off.

Combine bouillon cubes in boiling water and mix until well dissolved. Brush over turkey.

Roast at 325° for 3½ hours or until tender and juices run clear when thigh is pricked with a fork. Serves 24.

Contains 7 grams of fat for each 3½ ounce serving.

JOANN LOWE'S HADDOCK FILETS

4 haddock filets   1 Tbsp. olive oil
2 Tbsp. lemon juice

Mix lemon juice and olive oil together; pour into skillet and heat. Place filets in pan and saute until brown on each side, about 5 minutes. Serves 4.

Contains 4 fat grams per 3½ ounce serving.

Note: Use only 1 tablespoon olive oil as olive oil contains 14 fat grams per tablespoon.

LOW-FAT FRIED CATFISH

4 catfish fillets (about 3½ oz.   Dried dill weed
   each)
4 Tbsp. low-fat Italian salad
   dressing

Brush both sides of fish with low-fat salad dressing. Sprinkle with dill weed. Saute in a nonstick skillet that has been sprayed with a non-fat cooking spray. Turn and brown on other side for about 4 minutes on each side or until fish flakes easily. Use more cooking spray if needed. Serves 4.

Contains 3½ fat grams per serving.

BAKED COD WITH VEGETABLES

1 or 2 whole cod (8 oz. each),   1 or 2 stalks celery, cut in 2 inch
   scaled and filleted   pieces
1 sliced onion

Saute onion and celery in a skillet sprayed with a nonstick cooking spray. Place vegetables in bottom of a pan sprayed with cooking spray.

Place fish on top of vegetables. Bake at 400°F. for <u>10 minutes per inch of thickness.</u> Serves 2 to 4.

Four ounces cod contains 1 fat gram.

GRILLED TUNA STEAKS

4 (6 oz.) yellow fin tuna steak (¾ inch thick), skinned

½ c. lime juice
1 minced garlic clove

Combine lime juice and garlic in an 8x8 inch glass baking dish. Add tuna. Cover and marinate for 3 hours in refrigerator, turning occasionally.

Grill over medium heat for 8 to 10 minutes on each side, basting often with the marinade. Serves 4.

Contains 2 fat grams per serving.

CAROLYN WARREN'S ORANGE SOLE

1 lb. sole fillets (about 3 oz. each)
1 Tbsp. canola oil

1 orange (juice and grated rind)

Place fillets in an 8x12 inch baking pan that has been sprayed with a nonstick cooking spray.

Cut orange in half and squeeze juice into a bowl. Grate 2 teaspoons rind and add to bowl. Stir in canola oil. Mix well and pour over fish. Bake at 350°F. for about 20 to 25 minutes or until fish flakes easily when tested with a fork. Serves 4.

Contains 4½ grams of fat per 3 ounce serving.

BAKED LEMON COD

2 lb. cod filets
2 or 3 Tbsp. freshly squeezed
   lemon juice

2 tsp. paprika

Sprinkle lemon juice over cod. Sprinkle with paprika and bake at 450°F. for 15 minutes or until fish flakes. Serves 6.

Contains 1 fat gram for each 4 ounce serving.

OAT-CRUSTED TROUT

4 brook trout fillets (3½ oz. each)
⅓ c. rolled oats

1 Tbsp. canola oil or olive oil

Rinse trout under cold water. Pat dry with paper towels.

Spread out oats on waxed paper and press fish down on them, coating both sides. Heat oil in a nonstick skillet that has been liberally sprayed with a non-fat, non-stick cooking spray. Cook trout for about 5 minutes on each side. Serves 4.

Contains 5.1 grams of fat per 3½ ounce serving.
Note: Rainbow trout has 11.4 grams of fat not counting the fat content of the oil. Brook trout is the better choice.

BROILED HADDOCK

4 haddock fillets (about 4 oz. each)
6 Tbsp. Italian dressing (lite, lowfat)

Corn flake crumbs, finely crushed

Dip haddock in Italian dressing, then roll in crumbs until coated. Place on a broiler pan and broil 10 minutes on each side or until brown and flakes easily. Serves 4.
Contains 1½ grams of fat per serving.

SOUTHWESTERN HALIBUT

4 halibut steaks (4 oz. each)
2 Tbsp. lemon juice

8 Tbsp. thick and chunky salsa

Sprinkle lemon juice over halibut and marinate in the refrigerator for 30 to 45 minutes.
To prepare, place 2 tablespoons salsa on each steak and broil until fish flakes easily when pierced with a fork. Serves 4.
Contains 3½ fat grams per each 4 ounce serving.

"FRIED" BREADED COD

4 cod fillets (4 oz. each)
½ c. Egg Beaters or other egg substitute

¼ c. finely crushed lowfat cracker crumbs

Rinse fish in cool water and pat dry with paper towels. Dip fish in egg substitute, then coat with lowfat or nonfat cracker crumbs. Allow fish to set for 4 to 5 minutes, then "fry" in nonfat cooking spray until golden brown on both sides. Add more cooking spray if needed. Serves 4.
Contains about 2 fat grams per serving.

POACHED CATFISH

2 lemons
1 lb. catfish frozen fillets, thawed (4 oz. each)

Mrs. Dash seasoning

Squeeze juice from 1 lemon and heat in skillet. Place fillets in lemon juice. Cover and poach for 3 to 8 minutes or until fish flakes easily when tested with a fork. Season with Mrs. Dash. Cut second lemon into wedges or slices and serve with fish. Serves 4.

Contains 3 fat grams per 4 ounce serving.

SOLE WITH YOGURT SAUCE

1 lb. sole fillets (3 oz. each)   ½ tsp. dill weed (or to taste)
1 c. low-fat plain yogurt

Saute fish in a nonstick skillet that has been sprayed with a nonfat cooking spray. Brown on both sides.

Mix yogurt with dill weed to taste. Pour over fish and heat. Serves 4.

Contains 2½ fat grams per serving.

Optional: Serve with lemon wedges.

BROILED SOLE DIJON

1 lemon, cut in 8 thin slices   8 tsp. Dijon mustard
4 sole fillets

Place 2 lemon slices under each sole fillet in a broiler pan that has been sprayed with a nonstick cooking spray. Spread 2 teaspoons of mustard over each fillet. Broil fish 4 to 6 inches from heat in a preheated broiler for 5 minutes or until topping is bubbly and brown and fish is opaque. Serves 4.

Contains 1½ fat grams per serving.

PAT MEYERS' DILL PICKLE ROAST

1 (3 lb.) eye of round beef roast   Dill pickles
Juice from 1 pt. jar dill pickles

Place roast in a pan which has a lid. Pour juice over roast. Cover with lid or foil and bake at 325°F. for about 3 to 3½ hours or until tender and done to your taste.

Serve pickles in a side dish with roast. Serves 12 to 16.

Contains 4 grams fat for each 3 ounce serving.

SWISS FLANK STEAK

1 (2 lb.) flank steak   1 (16 oz.) can stewed tomatoes
1 c. chopped onion

Trim all visible fat from steak. Saute onion until transparent in a skillet that is sprayed with a nonstick cooking spray. Use more spray if needed.

Place flank steak in a 9x13 inch pan that has been sprayed with a nonfat cooking spray. Pour tomatoes and onions over steak. Bake at 350°F. for 1½ hours or until tender and cooked to desired degree of doneness. Serves 6 to 8.

Contains 8 fat grams per 3½ ounce serving.

BEEF TENDERLOIN STEAKS

4 (4 oz.) beef tenderloin steaks   Black pepper
Seasoned salt

Place beef steaks on rack in broiler pan so surface of meat is 2 to 3 inches from heat. Broil 10 to 15 minutes for rare, turning once, or broil to desired degree of doneness. Season with salt and pepper. Serves 4.

Contains 9 grams of fat per serving.

DR. CARL GARRETT'S LOW-FAT CHILI

Dr. Carl Garret is the minister of Emmanuel Baptist Church, Overland Park, Kansas.

½ lb. ground sirloin steak   1 pkg. 15 bean soup mix, cooked
1 pkg. Williams chili mix

Wash beans. Pour into a pot and cover with water. Let beans soak overnight, then cook for 3 to 4 hours or until tender. Add more water when needed.

Brown ground sirloin. Crumble and drain. Cool meat. Place in a colander and run water over it to remove as much fat as possible. Remove all fat from skillet. Return defatted ground beef to skillet and stir in chili mix. Add cooked and drained beans and liquid. Heat on low for 30 minutes to 1 hour, stirring often. Serves 4.

Each 3 ounce beef serving contains 13½ fat grams.

EASY ROAST BEEF

1 (3 lb.) eye of round roast   1 chopped onion
1 Tbsp. Worcestershire sauce

Remove all visible fat. Place roast on a large piece of heavy-duty foil in a roasting pan. Place under broiler and broil until brown. Spread Worcestershire sauce over the top of the roast. Sprinkle with chopped onions. Wrap tightly in foil and bake at 400°F. for 2½ to 3½ hours. Serves 9 to 16.

Contains 4 grams for each 3 ounce serving.

ITALIAN POT ROAST

1 (3 lb.) eye of round beef roast   1 (15 oz.) can stewed tomatoes
1 pkg. spaghetti sauce mix

Trim all visible fat from beef. Brown roast in a skillet sprayed with a nonstick cooking spray. Brown on all sides, then place in a crock pot. Mix together spaghetti sauce mix and tomatoes and pour over meat. Cover and cook on LOW for 7 to 9 hours or until meat is tender. Slice and serve. Serves 10 to 12.
Suggestion: Serve over hot spaghetti.
Contains 4 fat grams for each 3 ounce serving.

ARIZONA CHILI BEEF

2 lb. lean boneless round steak   1 (10½ oz.) can beef bouillon
1 (10 oz.) can enchilada or taco   broth
  sauce

Trim all visible fat from meat. Cut beef into ½ inch cubes. Simmer beef in mixture of enchilada sauce and beef broth in a covered pan for 45 to 60 minutes or until tender. Serve over rice or with tortillas. Serves 8.
Contains 6 fat grams per 3 ounce serving.

JIM'S BARBECUED BEEF SANDWICH

2 oz. roasted eye-of-round beef,   1 French roll, cut in half and
  sliced thin   warmed
1 Tbsp. barbecue sauce

Heat beef in microwave. Warm roll in microwave.
Place beef on French roll. Drizzle barbecue sauce over it. Top with remaining half of roll. Serves 1.
Contains 3½ fat grams per serving.

ROASTED PORK TENDERLOIN

2 lb. extra lean pork tenderloin   Garlic powder
Dried sage

Trim all visible fat from pork. Place in a roasting pan. Sprinkle sage and garlic over tenderloin. Place in a preheated oven and roast at 325°F. for 1 hour and 20 minutes or until fork tender and cooked to desired degree of doneness. Serves 6.
Contains 5 grams of fat for each 3 ounce serving.

DANISH PORK ROAST

1 (3 lb.) roast loin of pork
Pitted prunes

Peeled apples, cut in chunks or
 slices

Trim all visible fat from pork roast.

Partly separate meat from rib and stuff with as many apple chunks and pitted prunes as you wish to use. Tie the meat together. Roast in a roaster at 325°F. for about 3 hours or until tender and to desired doneness. Serves 8 to 10.

Contains 8 fat grams for each 3 ounce serving.

JANE BALLARD'S PORK CHOPS

4 pork chops, trimmed of visible
 fat
4 Tbsp. prepared mustard

1 (10¾ oz.) can Healthy Request,
 low-fat chicken noodle soup

Brown pork chops on both sides in a nonstick skillet sprayed with nonfat cooking spray. Drain on paper towels. Spread mustard over chops on both sides, then place them in a lightly sprayed pan. Pour soup over pork and bake at 325°F. for 45 minutes to 1 hour or until done and fork tender. Serves 4.

Contains 8 fat grams for each pork chop.

ROAST LEG OF LAMB

1 (3 lb.) leg of lamb
3 garlic cloves, slivered

Lemon pepper

Make small slits in meat surface with a sharp knife, then insert garlic sliver in each slit. Place meat on a rack in a roasting pan. Sprinkle with lemon pepper.

Roast, uncovered, for 30 to 35 minutes per pound or until done and fork tender. Serves 10.

Contains 6 fat grams per serving.

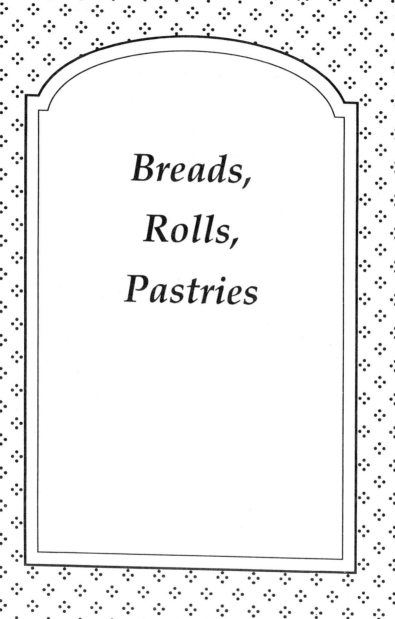

Breads,
Rolls,
Pastries

Anyway or anytime you serve them, breads, rolls and pastries are favorites. They are perfect morning, noon, or night, when served alone, or with a meal.

HOW TO

Quick breads are leavened with baking powder or baking soda. Mix lightly by hand. Overmixing will cause tough, coarse breads.

Yeast breads are leavened by yeast. Yeast is killed by using water that is too hot or too cold. Use liquid at 110° to 115°F. for standard mix (when yeast is dissolved in water) or 120°-130°F. for quick mix (when yeast is added with dry ingredients). Yeast breads are generally kneaded until smooth and elastic, about 8-10 minutes.

When making pie crust, measure very accurately and have the liquid well chilled. Handle the dough very little - if overworked, it will be tough.

TIMELY IDEAS

Quick rise yeast is readily available and does save rising time. Follow package directions for recipe changes that might be necessary.

Pie dough, pie crusts, or fruit pies can be frozen. Prepare cream pies or those with meringue just before serving and refrigerate.

YOUR CREATIVITY

Muffins are a popular quick bread. They can be sweet or savory, home-style or elegant. Add nuts, raisins, chocolate chips or fruit to the batter. Place jam in the center of the muffin before baking. Top with a streusel topping or seeds. Also, look to innovative whipped and flavored butters for a tasty treat.

New breads will liven up plain sandwiches. Try pita, egg buns, English muffins, Italian rolls or any of your other favorites.

Pies and pastries are not always sweet. Try cheese and egg tarts or quiche or puff pastry with a creamed seafood filling.

Applique a pie crust by cutting extra dough with a cookie cutter. Moisten and position on top of pie. Cut decorative slits for steam.

Serve pancakes or waffles with fruit, ice cream or whipped cream for dessert.

TIPS

Do not sift flour for baking bread or pies.

Breads become stale sooner if stored in the refrigerator; however, they will mold more quickly at room temperature.

For extra sheen, brush bread dough with an egg mixed before baking, or brush pie crust with milk and sprinkle with sugar before baking.

Remove bread, rolls or muffins from the pan quickly after baking to prevent the bottom crust from becoming too moist.

Store whole grain flour in the freezer to ensure freshness.

HOW MUCH?

While one roll, biscuit or muffin is a serving, many people will take two. Remember, serve plenty and freeze the remaining.

One (8 inch) pie will make 6 servings.

YOUR HEALTH

Foods rich in fiber are now recommended. This might be whole grain breads, including whole wheat, rye or pumpernickel breads, bran or oatmeal muffins, and corn bread from whole, ground corn meal.

The increased need for fiber does not mean an increase in your consumption of fat and calories. The calories and fat come from the butter, jams, or other spreads and these should be minimized.

When buying bread, read the label. Many "brown breads" are made from varying amounts of white flour and whole wheat flour. Check which flour is listed first, and note if colorings are added, or select "whole wheat" which must be made from 100% wholewheat flour.

BREADS, ROLLS, PASTRIES

ORANGE-BLUEBERRY MUFFINS

1 (13 oz.) pkg. light blueberry
  muffin mix
¼ c. egg substitute, slightly
  beaten

⅓ to ½ c. orange juice

Combine the 3 ingredients in a bowl and mix until moistened. Spoon into 12 muffin cups that have been sprayed with a nonfat cooking spray. Bake at 400°F. for 15 to 20 minutes or until golden brown. Cool in pan for 5 minutes before removing. Yield: 1 dozen.
Contains less than 1 fat gram per serving.

TESSA McKEE'S FAT-FREE CHEESE BISCUITS

2 c. Pioneer no-fat biscuit mix
¾ c. evaporated skim milk

½ c. fat free Cheddar cheese,
  grated

Combine biscuit mix, evaporated milk, and cheese in a bowl and mix. (If too dry, add 1 tablespoon evaporated skim milk at a time.) Spray a baking sheet with nonfat cooking spray and drop dough onto it. Bake at 425°F. for 10 to 12 minutes. Yield: 6 large biscuits or 12 small.
Contains no fat content unless you use reduced fat Bisquick mix.

JANE BALLARD'S CORN FLAKE PIE CRUST

3 c. corn flakes, crushed
1½ Tbsp. sugar

1½ Tbsp. lite or lowfat cream
  cheese

Crush corn flakes in a blender or a food processor. Mix in sugar, then add 1 tablespoon cream cheese and process. Add remaining ½ tablespoon cream cheese and process, blending well.
Spray a 9 inch pie pan with a nonfat cooking spray. Pour corn flake mixture into pan and press evenly over bottom and sides to form a crust. Chill 1 to 2 hours before adding filling. Yield: 1 pie crust.
Contains about 1 gram of fat per serving.

APPLE PANCAKES

2 c. lowfat pancake mix
⅓ c. applesauce

1 c. apple juice

Combine pancake mix, apple juice, and applesauce in a bowl and blend with a wire whisk. Batter may be slightly lumpy. Don't overmix.

Pour ¼ cup batter per pancake onto a griddle that has been heavily sprayed with a nonstick cooking spray and cook on both sides. Yield: 6 pancakes.

Contains about 2 fat grams per pancake.

PITA PIZZAS

1 pita bread
½ sliced tomato (about 3 to 4 slices)

½ oz. part-skim Mozzarella cheese, shredded

Heat pita in oven until hot and lightly browned. Remove from oven and top with sliced tomatoes. Sprinkle shredded Mozzarella cheese over the top. Return to oven or broiler and heat until cheese melts. Serves 1.

Contains 3 fat grams per serving.

GARLIC TOAST

1 loaf French bread, sliced
Butter-flavored cooking spray

Garlic salt

Place bread slices on a baking sheet that has been sprayed with butter-flavored cooking spray. Spray top of bread with butter-flavored spray. Sprinkle bread lightly with garlic salt. Bake at 375°F. for 8 to 10 minutes or until golden brown. Turn bread after 4 or 5 minutes, if desired, to brown both sides. Yield: 10 to 12 slices.

Contains 1 fat gram per slice.

CHEESE TOSTADOS

4 (6 inch) corn tortillas
¼ c. reduced-fat Cheddar cheese, shredded

½ c. thick and chunky salsa

Place tortillas on a nonstick baking sheet. Top with cheese. Bake at 350°F. until cheese melts and tortilla is crisp. (Optional: Top with slices of jalapeno.) Serve with chunky tomato salsa. Serves 4.

Note: Each tostado contains about 3 grams of fat.

ORANGE FRENCH TOAST

6 slices raisin bread
⅓ c. orange juice

½ c. egg substitute

Dip raisin bread into a mixture of orange juice and eggs. Fry on each side in pan sprayed with nonstick cooking spray. Serves 6.

Contains 1 gram of fat per slice.

TESSA'S EASY ROLLS

2 c. self-rising flour
¼ c. plus 2 Tbsp. lowfat
  mayonnaise

¼ c. nonfat buttermilk

Combine the 3 ingredients. Stir only until moistened. Spoon batter into muffin pans that have been sprayed with a nonstick vegetable cooking spray.

Bake at 375°F. for 12 to 15 minutes or until lightly browned. Makes 12 servings. Yield: 1 dozen rolls.

Contains 2 fat grams per serving.

CREPES

1 c. lowfat or nonfat baking mix
2 egg whites (or egg substitute)

1 c. skim milk

Combine the 3 ingredients and beat with a mixer until smooth. Spoon 2 tablespoons batter into a hot skillet that is generously sprayed with a nonstick cooking spray. Rotate skillet until batter thinly covers bottom of pan. Cook until brown. Turn and brown other side. Yield: 8 thin crepes.

Contains no fat grams if nonfat baking mix is used, about 1 fat gram per crepe if lowfat mix is used.

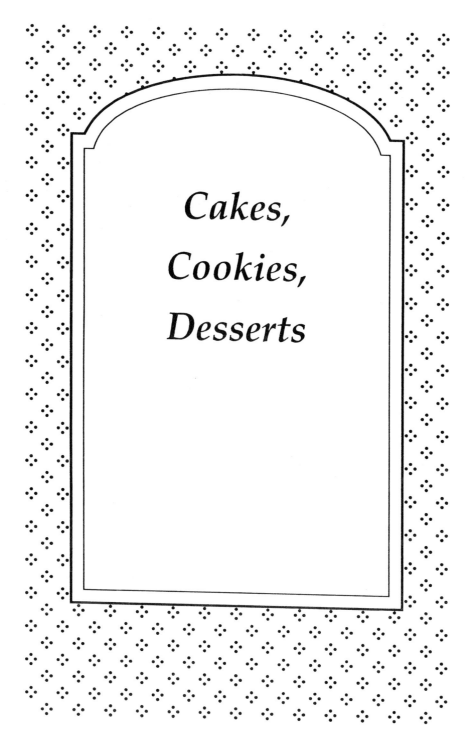

Cakes,
Cookies,
Desserts

Perhaps no food has more tradition than our cakes, cookies and desserts. Your favorite birthday cake, Grandma's favorite cookies, and that special holiday dessert are the foods that make memories.

HOW TO

When making cakes, cookies and desserts, be sure and measure accurately.

For best results, have ingredients at room temperature.

Cake pans should be greased with solid shortening, not oil or butter. Most are dusted with flour. Grease sheets for cookies only if directed.

Preheat the oven. Place pans in center of oven, not touching oven walls or other pans.

When blending dry and liquid ingredients, begin and end with the dry ingredients.

TIMELY IDEAS

Cookies freeze well, as you can freeze the baked cookies or the prepared dough. Cakes are best frozen before frosted. Do not freeze fluffy, boiled frosting or whipped cream frosting; these are best prepared just before serving. Be sure and keep cakes with whipped cream or cream cheese frosting refrigerated.

Keep a pound cake in the freezer, or a pound cake mix on the shelf. A dessert is only minutes away when pound cake is served with fruit, sauce or topping.

A frozen layered ice cream dessert or frozen fruit salad that can double as a dessert is a wonderful make-ahead dish when entertaining.

For a large party, dip ice cream into balls the day before and place on cookie sheet. Freeze until solid. Stack in a serving bowl and seal tightly with plastic wrap to prevent drying. Refreeze until serving time. The ice cream is a snap to serve.

YOUR CREATIVITY

Fun garnishes for a cake include chocolate curls, fresh berries, a drizzle of chocolate sauce over the frosting, coarsely chopped, toasted nuts or toasted coconut.

Ice cream, fruit, and a whipped topping, layered in tall glasses makes a beautiful, easy dessert.

TIPS

Sift cake flour. No need to sift all-purpose flour.

If you like soft, chewy cookies, bake only minimum time. Bake for the maximum time if crisp cookies are desired.

Store soft cookies in an airtight container. A slice of bread or apple will help keep them fresh. Store crisp cookies in a container with loose fitting lid.

HOW MUCH?

A layer cake serves 12 to 16.

One 9x13 inch pan gives 24 large or 48 small brownies or other bar cookies.

One serving of ice cream, or pudding is ½ cup. One-half gallon of ice cream makes 16 servings.

YOUR HEALTH

Select one whole-grain cookie, or a fruit dessert for the enjoyment without the guilt. Many times, this little sweet may be all that is needed to help you go on with a diet.

Save calories by using a low calorie, whipped topping and eliminate the icing on a cake.

A cheese and fruit tray is an elegant "help yourself" dessert and provides a relaxing, after meal treat, good nutrition, and no wasted calories.

Children love cookies so pack their cookies with nutrition. Select cookies made with cereal, then add raisins, nuts, shredded carrots, pumpkin, or fruits.

CAKES, COOKIES, DESSERTS

MYRTLE HULL'S APPLESAUCE ANGEL

1 angel food cake, baked and
  sliced
1 (15 oz.) can natural applesauce,
  chilled

Cinnamon

Slice angel food cake in 12 slices. Place cake slices on individual dessert dishes. Spoon chilled unsweetened natural applesauce over cake. Sprinkle with cinnamon. Serves 12.
Contains no fat grams!

DATE KISSES

2 egg whites
1 c. powdered sugar

1 c. chopped dates

Beat egg whites until stiff. Add sugar and dates. Drop from teaspoon onto pans sprayed with nonfat cooking spray and bake at 300°F. for about 10 to 12 minutes or until delicately browned. Cool. Store in tightly covered container. Yield: 2½ dozen.
Contains no fat!

VELORA HOLT'S MARSHMALLOW DROPS

2 c. Rice Krispies cereal
1 c. marshmallow cream

½ c. raisins

Heat marshmallow cream in top of a double boiler until syrupy. Remove from heat. Pour over cereal and raisins and mix well. Drop by teaspoonfuls onto aluminum foil. Refrigerate until firm. Yield: 3 dozen. Fat free.

Optional: Use corn flakes instead of Rice Krispies for a different taste.

GINGERBREAD-APPLESAUCE COOKIES

1 (14 oz.) pkg. gingerbread mix
⅓ c. applesauce

½ c. plain lowfat yogurt

Combine the 3 ingredients and mix until smooth. Drop teaspoonfuls of dough, about 2 inches apart, on greased cookie sheets and bake at 375°F. for 8 to 10 minutes or until firm. Yield: 4 dozen cookies.
Contains less than 1 fat gram each.

TONAH EBERHARDT'S PISTACHIO PUDDING

1 (4 oz.) pkg. lowfat, sugar-free
    instant pistachio pudding
    mix

2 c. plain nonfat yogurt
1 (20 oz.) can crushed pineapple
    and juice

Combine, mix, cover, and chill until serving time. Serves 4.
Contains about ½ fat gram per serving.

LOWFAT FUDGE BROWNIES

1 box lite fudge brownie mix
5.5 oz. Hershey's chocolate syrup

½ c. Egg Beaters

Combine all ingredients in a large mixing bowl and mix until moistened. If mixture is too dry, add a little water, 1 tablespoon at a time. Spray a 9x13 inch glass baking dish with nonfat cooking spray. Pour mixture into pan and bake at 350°F. for 25 to 30 minutes. Cool. Yield: 36 squares.
Contains 1½ grams fat per piece.

DOROTHY TOWNSEND'S MERINGUES

6 egg whites
¾ tsp. cream of tartar

⅔ c. sugar

Beat egg whites and cream of tartar at high speed of an electric mixer until soft peaks form. Stir in sugar, 1 tablespoon at a time, and beat until stiff peaks form.

Line 2 baking sheets with parchment paper. Draw 4 (4 inch) circles on each sheet of paper. Spoon meringue onto circles on paper and build up sides to form a shell or cup. Bake at 225°F. for 1 hour and 20 minutes. Turn oven off. Leave meringues in oven for 2 hours or overnight with oven doors closed. Don't open oven doors for at least 2 hours. Serves 8.

Contains no fat.

Fill meringues with chocolate pudding, sweetened strawberries, cherry pie filling, or filling of your choice.

CHERRY DUMP CAKE

1 (21 oz.) can lite cherry pie filling
1 box white or yellow light cake
    mix

1 c. liquid Butter Buds

Mix 2 packets Butter Buds with 1 cup water for liquid Butter Buds.

CAKES, COOKIES, DESSERTS

MYRTLE HULL'S APPLESAUCE ANGEL

1 angel food cake, baked and   Cinnamon
   sliced
1 (15 oz.) can natural applesauce,
   chilled

      Slice angel food cake in 12 slices. Place cake slices on individual dessert dishes. Spoon chilled unsweetened natural applesauce over cake. Sprinkle with cinnamon. Serves 12.
      Contains no fat grams!

DATE KISSES

2 egg whites   1 c. chopped dates
1 c. powdered sugar

      Beat egg whites until stiff. Add sugar and dates. Drop from teaspoon onto pans sprayed with nonfat cooking spray and bake at 300°F. for about 10 to 12 minutes or until delicately browned. Cool. Store in tightly covered container. Yield: 2½ dozen.
      Contains no fat!

VELORA HOLT'S MARSHMALLOW DROPS

2 c. Rice Krispies cereal   ½ c. raisins
1 c. marshmallow cream

      Heat marshmallow cream in top of a double boiler until syrupy. Remove from heat. Pour over cereal and raisins and mix well. Drop by teaspoonfuls onto aluminum foil. Refrigerate until firm. Yield: 3 dozen. Fat free.
      Optional: Use corn flakes instead of Rice Krispies for a different taste.

GINGERBREAD-APPLESAUCE COOKIES

1 (14 oz.) pkg. gingerbread mix   ½ c. plain lowfat yogurt
⅓ c. applesauce

      Combine the 3 ingredients and mix until smooth. Drop teaspoonfuls of dough, about 2 inches apart, on greased cookie sheets and bake at 375°F. for 8 to 10 minutes or until firm. Yield: 4 dozen cookies.
      Contains less than 1 fat gram each.

TONAH EBERHARDT'S PISTACHIO PUDDING

1 (4 oz.) pkg. lowfat, sugar-free instant pistachio pudding mix

2 c. plain nonfat yogurt
1 (20 oz.) can crushed pineapple and juice

Combine, mix, cover, and chill until serving time. Serves 4. Contains about ½ fat gram per serving.

LOWFAT FUDGE BROWNIES

1 box lite fudge brownie mix
5.5 oz. Hershey's chocolate syrup

½ c. Egg Beaters

Combine all ingredients in a large mixing bowl and mix until moistened. If mixture is too dry, add a little water, 1 tablespoon at a time. Spray a 9x13 inch glass baking dish with nonfat cooking spray. Pour mixture into pan and bake at 350°F. for 25 to 30 minutes. Cool. Yield: 36 squares.

Contains 1½ grams fat per piece.

DOROTHY TOWNSEND'S MERINGUES

6 egg whites
¾ tsp. cream of tartar

⅔ c. sugar

Beat egg whites and cream of tartar at high speed of an electric mixer until soft peaks form. Stir in sugar, 1 tablespoon at a time, and beat until stiff peaks form.

Line 2 baking sheets with parchment paper. Draw 4 (4 inch) circles on each sheet of paper. Spoon meringue onto circles on paper and build up sides to form a shell or cup. Bake at 225°F. for 1 hour and 20 minutes. Turn oven off. Leave meringues in oven for 2 hours or overnight with oven doors closed. Don't open oven doors for at least 2 hours. Serves 8.

Contains no fat.

Fill meringues with chocolate pudding, sweetened strawberries, cherry pie filling, or filling of your choice.

CHERRY DUMP CAKE

1 (21 oz.) can lite cherry pie filling
1 box white or yellow light cake mix

1 c. liquid Butter Buds

Mix 2 packets Butter Buds with 1 cup water for liquid Butter Buds.

Spray 9x11 inch Pyrex dish with a nonstick cooking spray. Spread cherries evenly in bottom of pan. Sprinkle dry cake mix over top of fruit. Pour liquid Butter Buds over top. Bake at 350°F. for 35 to 40 minutes or until golden brown. Serves 24.

Contains 1½ grams fat per serving.

BETTY KOLBE'S CHOCOLATE APPLESAUCE CAKE

1 box low-fat chocolate cake mix
1 (16 oz.) can applesauce

½ to ¾ c. Egg Beaters egg
   substitute

Combine the 3 ingredients in a mixing bowl and mix until well-blended. Pour into a 9x13 inch pan that was sprayed with a nonfat cooking spray. Bake as package directs. Serves 12 to 16.

Contains less than ½ fat gram per serving.

CHERRY ANGEL JUBILEE

1 angel food cake
¾ c. currant jelly

1 (16 oz.) can pitted Bing cherries,
   drained

Cut cake into 12 wedges.

In a skillet, melt currant jelly with drained Bing cherries. Heat until hot and simmering.

Place cake wedge on individual dessert plates. Spoon cherry mixture over it. Serves 12.

Contains no fat grams.

PEACH TRIFLE

1 (11½ oz.) Entenmann's fat free
   pound cake
1 pkg. non-fat vanilla pudding

1 pt. fresh peaches, peeled and
   cubed

Cut pound cake into ½ inch slices. Reserve 5 slices. Arrange remaining slices in bottom of a 2½ quart glass bowl.

Prepare pudding as package directs, then spoon pudding over cake. Cover with chopped peaches. Place remaining 5 slices in star shape on top of fruit. Serves 6.

Contains no fat grams!

MYRTLE HULL'S STRAWBERRY DESSERT

⅓ c. frozen strawberries
1 c. lowfat vanilla frozen yogurt

½ c. crushed ice or 6 ice cubes

Crush ice cubes in blender until slushy. Remove ice and reserve. Blend berries and frozen yogurt in the blender container until smooth. Add crushed ice and mix until blended. Serve in sherbet dishes. Serves 2.

Contains 1 fat gram per serving.

ANGEL BANANA PUDDING

½ angel food cake (loaf size)
1 small box fat-free banana
  pudding mix

2 to 3 bananas, peeled and sliced

Slice angel food cake and place in bottom of a dessert bowl.

Prepare banana pudding mix as package directs. Cool. Spread ½ of pudding over angel food cake. Top with 1 or 2 sliced bananas.

Repeat layers, ending with pudding on top. Serves 4.

Contains 1 fat gram per serving.

Note: Angel food cakes require no fat and they are made with egg whites.

YOGURT BROWNIES

1 pkg. Duncan Hines lowfat
  fudge brownie mix

⅓ c. low-fat plain yogurt
2 egg whites, lightly beaten

Combine brownie mix, yogurt, and 2 egg whites in a bowl and mix until blended. Pour mixture into a 9x13 inch pan that has been sprayed with a nonstick cooking spray. Bake at 350°F. for about 23 to 25 minutes or until cake tests done. Cool. Cut into squares. Yield: 24 brownies.

Contains about 2 fat grams per serving.

LOUISE HOLTZINGER'S WAFFLE SUNDAE

1 pkg. frozen waffles (low-fat)
1 small pkg. frozen sliced
  strawberries

Fat free ice cream

Toast or bake waffles. Cool. Thaw strawberries. Place a waffle on a dessert plate. Top with 1 scoop fat free ice cream. Spoon thawed berries over ice cream. Repeat with number of people you are serving.

Contains 2½ grams per serving.

Optional: Spoon berries over a toasted waffle and top with 1 teaspoon low calorie whipped topping.

Note: There are now round miniature frozen waffles on the market.

ANGEL SHORTCAKES

1 box angel food cake mix
1 (10 oz.) pkg. frozen, sliced,
  sweetened strawberries

1 (6 Tbsp.) ctn. low-fat whipped
  topping

Prepare angel food cake mix as directed on package. Drop ½ cup mixture onto a cookie sheet that has been sprayed with a nonstick cooking spray. Drop ½ cup of mixture 2 inches apart. Put 6 inch shortcakes on each cookie sheet. Bake at 375°F. for 10 to 15 minutes. Remove immediately. Repeat until all batter is used. Split shortcakes and top with berries. Place top part of cake over berries and spoon more berries over. Garnish with 1 tablespoon whipped topping.
Contains 1 fat gram per serving.

DOROTHY TOWNSEND'S CHOCOLATE FROSTING

1 env. Dream Whip
½ c. skim milk, chilled

1 (2 oz.) pkg. lowfat, sugar-free
  chocolate pudding mix

Blend Dream Whip and milk together and beat until stiff. Add pudding mix and beat until light and fluffy. (Add more milk if mixture is too thick.)
Frost angel food cakes or low-fat cakes and brownies. Yield: 2½ cups.
Contains ½ fat gram per tablespoon.

APRICOT CAKE

1 pkg. lowfat yellow cake mix
1 or 2 (16 oz.) cans apricots,
  chopped and drained

4 egg whites or ½ c. Egg Beaters

Combine all ingredients in a mixer bowl and beat with an electric mixer until well blended. Spray a 9x13 inch pan with a nonstick cooking spray. Spread batter in prepared pan and bake at 350°F. for 30 minutes or until done. Cut into squares. Serves 12.
Contains 2 fat grams per serving.
Optional: Place cake square in a dessert plate and spoon heated apricot preserves over it.

ORANGE SNAPS

1 (11 oz.) can mandarin oranges,
  drained
1 (8 oz.) ctn. nonfat cream cheese,
  softened

Gingersnaps

Finely chop oranges. Whip cream cheese, then stir in finely chopped oranges. Spread mixture on gingersnaps. Yield: 1 cup.

Contains about 1 fat gram per cookie.

Optional: If needed, sweeten with powdered sugar to taste. If too thick, add a small amount of juice from oranges.

VELORA HOLT'S STRAWBERRY ICE CREAM

⅔ c. evaporated skim milk (1 small can)
1 (10 oz.) pkg. frozen strawberries, thawed

¼ c. sugar

Chill milk in ice tray until almost frozen at edges.

Mix ice cold milk in a cold 1½ quart bowl of electric mixer, using cold beaters. Whip at high speed until stiff.

Combine strawberries and sugar when milk is in freezer. Gradually add strawberry mixture to whipped skim milk. Beat at low speed until well mixed. Freeze until firm, about 3 hours. Serves 6 to 8.

Contains no fat!

GRAHAM CRACKER CRUST

16 small graham crackers, crushed to equal 1 c.
3 Tbsp. Butter Buds liquid

¾ tsp. liquid sweetener or 1 tsp. sugar

Prepare Butter Buds as package directs.

Combine all ingredients, mix well, and press firmly into a 9 inch pie plate. Bake 8 to 10 minutes at 350°F. Refrigerate before filling. Yield: 1 crust.

Contains 4 fat grams.

STRAWBERRY PINEAPPLE SHERBET

1 pt. fresh strawberries, sliced
1 (8 oz.) can crushed pineapple and juice

1 (6 oz.) can frozen pineapple juice concentrate (do not dilute)

Combine all ingredients in blender and blend for 2 minutes. Pour into 4 to 6 sherbet dishes and freeze.

Let set at room temperature for 20 to 25 minutes before serving. Serves 4 to 6.

Contains about ½ fat gram per serving.

LEMON GLAZED CAKE

2 c. powdered sugar
Juice from 2 lemons (or 4 Tbsp.
  lemon juice)

Non-fat pound cake or angel
  food cake

Combine the sugar and lemon juice and mix until well blended.
Use this icing on Entenmann's lowfat pound cake or angel food
cake. Heat cake. While cake is hot, poke holes with fork and pour icing
over top. Serves 8 to 10.
Contains no fat grams.

VELMA STEWART'S FRESH BERRY TOPPING

1 c. fresh berries (your choice)
2½ Tbsp. honey

½ c. non-fat plain yogurt

You may use your choice of strawberries, raspberries, blackberries,
or blueberries, etc.
In a medium bowl, crush berries. Stir in honey and mix well. Combine berry mixture with yogurt.
This topping can be spooned over fat free pound cake, angel food
cake, or fat free ice cream. This mixture could also be used over waffles or
pancakes. Yield: 1½ cups.
Contains no fat grams.

MOTHER'S BAKED CINNAMON APPLES

6 to 8 cooking apples
1 (9 oz.) pkg. red hot cinnamon
  candies

Water

Wash and core apples. Use a fork to prick tops of each of the apples,
then randomly prick body of each apple several times.
Place apples in a baking dish that was sprayed with a non-fat
cooking spray. Fill center of each apple with about 2 tablespoons of "red
hots" candies.
Pour ½ inch water around apples. Bake at 350°F. for about 45 minutes or until tender. Serves 6 to 8.
Contains no fat.

EASY FRUIT DESSERT

3 bananas, sliced
15 fresh strawberries, rinsed and
  sliced

Cool Whip whipped topping
  (lite)

Put equal amounts of bananas and strawberries into 4 dessert dishes. Top each with a dollop of whipped topping. Serves 4.

Contains 1 gram of fat per serving.

CRUNCHY ANGEL FOOD CAKE

1 pkg. Betty Crocker 1-step angel
  food cake mix
¾ c. coarsely crushed Wheaties
  or Total cereal

½ tsp. cinnamon

Mix cereal and cinnamon. Prepare cake mix as package directs, except fold cereal mixture into batter. Pour into a Bundt cake pan that was sprayed with Pam cooking spray. Bake and cool as directed on package. Serves 12.

Contains no fat grams!

BANANA-PINEAPPLE SHERBET

1½ c. evaporated skim milk
2 bananas, mashed

1 (20 oz.) can crushed pineapple,
  drained

Chill the milk and beaters in a mixing bowl in the freezer when ice crystals form around the edge of the milk. Whip it with an electric mixer until it stands in stiff peaks. Stir in mashed bananas and drained pineapple. Freeze for 30 minutes or until firm, then whip again. Cover and return to freezer until ready to serve. Serves 6.

Contains ½ fat gram per serving.

PINEAPPLE YOGURT PUDDING

1 large pkg. instant non-fat
  vanilla pudding

1 (16 oz.) ctn. plain nonfat yogurt
1 (20 oz.) can crushed pineapple

Mix all ingredients together. Cover and refrigerate several hours or overnight.

Note: The pudding is mixed in dry. Do not mix pudding as package directs. Serves 6 to 8.

Contains no fat grams.

PINEAPPLE CAKE

1 yellow low-fat cake mix,
  prepared
1 (20 oz.) can crushed pineapple,
  drained

Lowfat or nonfat whipped
  topping

Prepare cake as package directs, then stir in pineapple. Pour into a 9x13 inch pan that has been sprayed with a nonfat cooking spray and bake as directed on package. Cool.

Frost with Cool Whip lowfat whipped topping. Cut into squares and serve. Serves 24.

Contains about 2 fat grams per serving.

Optional: Stir a can of crushed and drained pineapple into the whipped topping, then frost the cooled cake. Or, spoon pineapple over frosted cake.

PINEAPPLE PUDDING

1 small box fat free vanilla
   pudding
1 (20 oz.) can crushed pineapple,
   drained

1 box vanilla wafers

Mix pudding as directed on package. Place a layer of vanilla wafers on bottom of a bowl, then a layer of pineapple and a layer of pudding. Repeat layers. Refrigerate for 2 hours before serving. Serves 6.

Contains about 2 grams of fat per serving.

FROZEN FRUIT SLUSH

2 c. strawberries, sliced
2 c. sliced bananas

1 (12 oz.) can ginger ale

Combine all ingredients. Mix and freeze to a mush. Divide into portions and serve. Serves 4.

Contains less than 1 fat gram per serving.

FROZEN STRAWBERRY YOGURT

2 c. fresh strawberries or 1 (10
   oz.) pkg. frozen berries,
   thawed

1 c. non-fat plain yogurt
$\frac{1}{3}$ c. confectioners sugar

Puree berries. Add sugar and yogurt and process until well blended. Optional: Stir in 1 tablespoon lemon juice.

Pour into ice trays or ice cream machine and freeze according to manufacturer's directions. Serves 4.

Contains negligible fat gram.

VANILLA RICE PUDDING

1 small pkg. vanilla non-fat
   pudding mix (not instant)

$\frac{1}{2}$ c. Minute rice
$\frac{2}{3}$ c. raisins

Prepare pudding mix according to directions on the box, using skim milk.

Cook rice as package directs.

Combine pudding, rice, and raisins and mix well. Serves 4.

Contains no fat!

Optional: Stir in ¼ teaspoon cinnamon and ⅛ teaspoon nutmeg.

CHOCOLATE-BANANA ANGEL FOOD CAKE

1 loaf size angel food cake, baked   Chocolate syrup
2 to 4 sliced bananas

Slice angel food cake and place slices on individual desert dishes. Top with sliced bananas. Drizzle 2 tablespoons chocolate syrup over each serving of bananas and cake. Serves 6 to 8.

Contains 0.4 fat gram per serving (about ½ gram).

APRICOT SQUARES

1 pkg. angel food cake mix (must   1 (21 oz.) can apricot pie filling
   use 1-step mix)   Powdered sugar

Combine cake mix with pie filling and spread in a 10x15 inch jellyroll pan that had been sprayed with a nonstick cooking spray.

Bake at 350°F. for 15 to 20 minutes or until lightly browned. Cool. Cut into squares.

Sprinkle with sifted powdered sugar. Serves 40.

Contains no fat grams per serving.

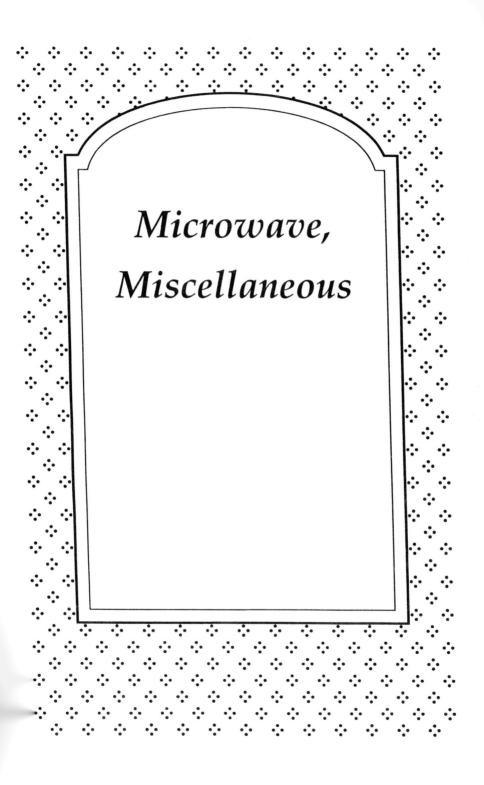

Microwave,
Miscellaneous

The microwave oven really has revolutionized how many people cook. It is used for family meals, gourmet cooking, and many extras that make meal planning fun and easy.

HOW TO

Each brand or type of microwave oven varies. Commonly their cooking wattage ranges from about 450 to 700 or more and this means wide differences in cooking times. Generally begin with the minimum cooking time, then add more time, in small amounts, as needed to complete the cooking. Check progress frequently.

While some microwave ovens have only one basic setting, others have 10 or more. HIGH or "100%" power is used the most frequently. Lower power settings are used for dense or delicate foods or other special cooking needs.

Standing time is simply time to allow the food to finish cooking. Removing food from the oven just a little before it is done may be difficult to remember, but it is important, since cooking time can always be added.

Arrange foods with larger, denser portions to the outside of the plate for even cooking. Other tips for even cooking include using round dishes instead of square and selecting a ring mold when cooking a food that cannot be stirred.

TIMELY IDEAS

Microwave cooking is quick and it will trim time from meal preparation. The microwave oven also lets you handle your time better.

Quick defrosting is a definite plus for the microwave. Generally turn the cooking power down to about 30% or a defrost cycle. If you have only a HIGH (100%) power setting, alternate between short cooking and standing cycles until the food is thawed.

Leftovers are now both tasty and time-saving. Make extra and freeze for busier evenings ahead. Just thaw and heat in the microwave oven.

Cooking and serving in one dish is a definite microwave plus since you save clean-up time.

YOUR CREATIVITY

Tasks that are easy for the microwave oven may spark your creativity. Heat syrup or toppings for ice cream or pancakes, melt chocolate chips to drizzle over a frosted cake or dazzle your family with quick, warm drinks.

Speed up cooking out on the barbecue grill but keep all of the flavor. Partially cook the food in the microwave oven. Then transfer to the hot grill and quickly finish cooking.

TIPS

It is easy to know what to cover food with if you think about the cover itself. Paper towels absorb moisture and are especially helpful when heating rolls or other crisp food. Wax paper is a loose cover and helps prevent splattering. Plastic wrap forms a tight seal which retains moisture.

Some tips are helpful if you wish the food to appear more browned. Many colorful sauces are perfect, including soy, teriyaki or sweet and sour sauces, jam, jelly or catsup. Crushed chips, bread crumbs, chopped nuts, crisp bacon, or shredded cheese may also add color.

YOUR HEALTH

Microwave ground beef in a colander so the fat drains off. Set colander inside a glass pie plate. Microwave, stirring frequently, until done.

A microwave oven is perfect when the dilemma arises that only one in the family is on a diet. Cooking single servings of any special dietary food is quick and easy.

A trip to the fast food restaurant may not provide you with the most nutrition, even when you are in a hurry. Instead, think about the microwave oven. Keep single servings of chicken pieces, fish fillets, or other favorites handy in the freezer. A few minutes of microwave cooking is all that is needed for a quick meal that offers the best nutrition.

MICROWAVE, MISCELLANEOUS

MICROWAVE TURKEY BREAST

1 (2 lb.) turkey breast, skinned   Paprika
Nonfat butter cooking spray

Remove all visible fat from skinned turkey breast. Wash with cold water and pat dry with paper towels. Spray exterior with nonfat butter cooking spray. Sprinkle with paprika. Place breast side down and cook on FULL power for 12 to 15 minutes. Turn turkey 4 times during cooking, every 3 to 4 minutes.

Remove from microwave, cover with tent of foil, and let set for 15 minutes. Serves 8.

Contains 3 fat grams per 3½ ounce serving.

MICROWAVE RASPBERRY SAUCE

1 (10 oz.) pkg. frozen raspberries   1 tsp. lemon juice
2 tsp. cornstarch

Place frozen berries in a 4 cup glass measuring cup. Push DEFROST and cook 3 to 3½ minutes or until thawed. Drain juice, but reserve.

Combine cornstarch with 1 tablespoon of raspberry juice and mix to form a paste. Stir in remaining raspberry juice. Stir in berries and cook for 6 minutes. Stir once every minute. Add lemon juice and mix. Refrigerate. Serve chilled over nonfat ice cream or angel food cake. Yield: ¾ cup.

Contains no fat!

GERI KIRCH'S SPANISH RICE

½ lb. extra lean hamburger   1½ c. Minute rice
1 or 2 (14½ oz.) cans stewed
   tomatoes with onion

Brown the hamburger in a skillet. Crumble and drain on paper towels. Pour into colander and rinse off fat.

Remove all fat from skillet. Return hamburger meat to skillet. Stir in tomatoes and mix together. Heat well. Add rice mix and heat until hot. Season to taste. Serves 3 to 4.

Contains 14 fat grams for each 3 ounce serving.

STRAWBERRY YOGURT POPSICLES

1 (16 oz.) pkg. frozen
  strawberries, crushed
1 (8 oz.) ctn. strawberry low-fat
  yogurt

⅔ c. cranberry juice

Thaw and crush strawberries. Combine the 3 ingredients in a bowl and mix well. Spoon evenly into paper cups. Insert a wooden stick into the center of each cup and freeze until firm. Yield: 10 servings.

Contains negligible fat grams (less than ½ fat gram per serving).

PARMESAN CHEESE POPCORN

8 to 10 c. air-popped popcorn
Butter-flavored cooking spray

⅓ c. fat-free Parmesan cheese

Pour popcorn into a bowl. Spray well with butter flavored spray. Sprinkle with Parmesan and toss to mix. Repeat process until popcorn is coated with butter spray and nonfat Parmesan cheese. Makes 4 servings.

Contains about 1 gram per serving.

YERBA BUENA TEA

1 c. water
3 fresh mint leaves

1 Tbsp. skim milk

Bring 1 cup water to a boil in a small saucepan. Add 3 fresh mint leaves. Turn off heat. Let it steep or set for 3 minutes. Pour into a cup and stir in skim milk. Serves 1.

Contains no fat grams.

Note: "Yerba Buena" means good herb. This is a healthy tea to which some people contribute their longevity (according to my Uncle Richard Bennett who contributed this recipe).

BASIC LOWFAT WHITE SAUCE

2 c. skim milk
3 Tbsp. flour

1 packet Butter Buds mix

Do not dilute Butter Buds.

Combine flour, milk, and Butter Buds in a saucepan and mix well. Heat, stirring constantly, until thickened. Season if desired. Yield: 2 cups.

ALFALFA SPROUTS

1 Tbsp. alfalfa sprouts
1 widemouthed qt. jar (glass)

Water

Place alfalfa seeds in the clear glass jar. Cover with water and soak overnight at room temperature.

Pour off water, rinse seeds, and drain well. Place jar on its side in a dark place, but at room temperature. Repeat process each morning. Seeds will start to sprout in 2 or 3 days. Rinsing removes hulls and prevents souring. Allow 6 to 7 days for sprouts growth. The last 2 days, sprouts should be placed in indirect light to develop chlorophyll. Makes 6 servings.

Contains <u>no fat.</u>

Note: Sprouts are good on sandwiches and salads.

"TONIC" FOR HEALTHY PLANTS

1 env. Knox unflavored gelatine   3 c. cold water
1 c. hot water

Dissolve gelatine in 1 cup hot water. Mix well. Stir in 3 cups cold water. Pour into jar with tight lid. Use once monthly on your plants. They will be healthier and greener. Yield: 4 cups.

INDEX OF RECIPES

You are what you eat. There is no denying it. Most people want to feel good, be energetic, and enjoy life. Most want to be trim no matter what their bone structure. In addition, most people want to enjoy the food they eat, and not spend every moment on some ridiculous diet.

The key to this well-being is good nutrition, found in the foods you eat. It is not found in eating just one miracle food. Instead, it is found in all the foods you eat. It is not based on just what you eat today, or next week, or next year. Wellness is a lifetime of proper eating and choices.

But what are the right choices? If you think the "right food" is boring, "rabbit" food, you couldn't be more wrong. There is real variety and a world of good food when you eat for wellness. And to help you, the United States Department of Agriculture, Human Nutrition Information Service has outlined some simple guidelines to lead you toward wise food choices.

The current guidelines are:

Eat a variety of foods.

Maintain desirable weight.

Avoid too much fat, saturated fat, and cholesterol.

Eat foods with adequate starch and fiber.

Avoid too much sugar.

Avoid too much sodium.

These guidelines are as simple and as basic as they seem. Let's explore some of them more.

EAT A VARIETY OF FOODS

You need more than 40 different nutrients for good health. These include vitamins, minerals, protein, fat, carbohydrates, and water. No one food contains all the nutrients needed, so it is important to eat a variety of foods each day.

To make the selections easier, the foods are divided into major food groups. The major food groups and the servings recommended by the USDA, for each are as follows:

Food Category	Servings Per Day
Breads, Cereals and other grain products including whole-grain foods)	6-11 (include several servings of whole-grain products daily)
Fruits	2-4
Vegetables	3-5
Meat, Poultry, Fish (or alternates like eggs, dry beans, nuts, and seeds)	2-3 (total of 5-7 ounces lean)
Milk, Cheese and Dairy	2 servings
Fats, Sweets	Avoid too many fats and sweets.

Be sure to select different foods within each group. For example, eating an apple is a wise food choice, but eating 4 each day, without selecting any other fruits, does not provide the needed nutrients.

MAINTAIN DESIRABLE WEIGHT

If you are overweight, or have ever thought about dieting, you might have been skeptical when you read the list above. However, eating a variety of foods does not prevent weight loss.

Losing weight does mean that you have to choose the variety of foods eaten even more carefully. The best diet is one that provides a variety of foods and supplies all of the nutrients needed, while it eliminates or reduces the foods that supply just calories like sugars, sweets, fats, soft drinks, and other calorie-rich foods. Eating a variety of foods, and even several servings each day of fruits, vegetables and whole-grain breads and cereals will provide all of the nutrients you need. If you select these foods carefully, and avoid high-calorie choices, you will be able to lose weight and keep it off.

Some tips to cut calories without cutting nutrition include:

AVOID SECOND SERVINGS. Gradually cut back on serving size.

USE LOWER-CALORIE VERSIONS OF THE FOOD. Select low-fat dairy products, or fruits packed without sugar. Learn to make substitutions for lowering calories, like low-fat yogurt for sour cream.

LIMIT HIGH-CALORIE BEVERAGES.

LEARN LOW-CALORIE COOKING TECHNIQUES. Roast, broil, boil, steam or poach foods. Avoid frying.

SELECT LEAN CUTS OF MEAT. Trim visible fat and remove the skin from chicken and fish.

AVOID BUTTER, MARGARINE, SAUCES, OR GRAVY. Use spices, herbs, lemon-juice, or other low-calorie seasonings.

KNOW WHAT "ONE SERVING" REALLY IS. Breads and cereals: One slice of bread, ½ hamburger bun, ½ cup rice or pasta, or 1 ounce of cereal (one oversized muffin may actually count as 2 servings.)

Fruit: One, medium whole fruit, ½ cup canned fruit, or ¾ cup juice.

Vegetables: ½ cup cooked or 1 cup of leafy, raw vegetables.

Meat: 5 to 7 ounces of lean meat. Count ½ cup cooked dry beans or 2 tablespoons of peanut butter as 1 ounce of meat.

Milk, dairy: 1 cup milk, 8 ounces yogurt, 1½ ounces natural cheese, 2 ounces process cheese.

ACTIVITY HELPS LEAD TO WEIGHT LOSS. The basics of weight loss go beyond the right food choices. For real weight loss, you must use more calories than you consume. To lose one pound you must use 3500 calories more than you consume.

But how is it possible to use up more calories than you consume, and still eat the variety of foods that your body needs? The key is activity or exercise.

You say exercise is not for you? Well, some types of exercise may be just for a few, very fit athletes. However, most people can add some activity to their lifestyle. These activities, added at a slow, even pace will soon make a real difference in your fitness program. Some changes are hardly called exercise at all — they are just routine changes, like walking instead of riding. Others are exercise. Remember, whether it is exercise or just activity, the number of calories burned depends on the degree of activity and the length of time the activity is done.

Set goals, and start right now. There will never be a better time. Remember, before you start with a sport or exercise program and new diet, check first with your doctor.

Walking is one of the easiest ways to burn calories. A quiet walk burns twice as many calories as standing still. Walk briskly and you will burn three times as many. And walking briskly for ½ hour each day (without eating more food) can result in a loss of 17 pounds each year.

Add more stretching, bending, and overall activity to all of your chores. Cleaning house burns 125-310 calories per hour. Scrubbing floors, or weeding gardens burns 315-480 calories per hour or the same as jogging, or playing tennis. Hard work, such as shoveling snow, spading gardens, aerobic dancing, swimming, or chopping wood burns 480-625 calories per hour.

Many people may find it simple to use the stairs instead of the elevator, park further away from the mall, take several 1-minute stretch breaks during the day, go dancing, or join a community sports league.

Another added benefit of exercise is that it may help relieve tension and tension may lead to overeating.

AVOID TOO MUCH FAT, SATURATED FAT, AND CHOLESTEROL

Recommendations for the U.S. population as a whole are to reduce the amount of fat, saturated fat and cholesterol in the diet.

Fat is a nutrient. It is the most concentrated source of calories, since it provides 9 calories per gram, while protein and carbohydrates provide 4 calories per gram.

Cholesterol is a fat-like substance found in the cells of humans and animals. It is needed to form hormones and other body substances, and the body is able to make the cholesterol it needs. It is found in meat, poultry, fish, milk and egg yolks. Cholesterol is not found in plant foods like fruits and vegetables.

Today, about 40% of the calories in a typical U.S. diet come from fat. Recommendations are to reduce this to about 30%-35%. But how?

SELECT LOW-FAT DAIRY PRODUCTS.

SELECT LEAN MEATS. (Remember, reduce fat by trimming the fat from meat and removing the skin of poultry. However, both the lean and fat of meat and the meat and skin of poultry contain cholesterol.)

CAREFULLY SELECT YOUR PREPARATION METHOD. Avoid frying or deep frying.

REDUCE THE FAT ADDED WHEN EATING. Prime sources are salad dressing, sour cream, butter, gravy, and other extras added when eating.

EAT FOODS WITH ADEQUATE STARCH AND FIBER. Carbohydrates supply sugar and starch. Sugar usually contains only calories, while starches are good sources of vitamins and minerals.

Fiber refers to the parts of plant foods which are not digestible by humans. Different types of fiber have different functions. It is not clear exactly how much and what types of fiber we need in the diet. However, most Americans should increase their consumption of fiber-containing food.

Foods that are good sources of fiber and starch are whole-grain breads and cereals, fruits, vegetables, dry beans and peas.

AVOID TOO MUCH SUGAR

Too much sugar is directly linked to tooth decay. Another key fact is that sugar provides calories - but the calories are "empty" or lacking other important nutrients. Frequently, eating sugary foods means that you are not eating enough of the foods that provide the needed nutrients.

When considering your sugar intake, don't just think of the sugar bowl. Remember also the brown sugar in baking, the corn syrup, honey and molasses used as toppings or ingredients. Sure the sweet candy or soda and the rich desserts like cakes, pies and cookies contain sugar, but don't forget other sugar sources, like syrup on pancakes, some salads, breakfast rolls, coffee cakes, streusel-topped muffins, jams, jelly, and a host of other sugary foods.

Sugar can be reduced in your everyday diet. Perhaps these hints will help.

READ THE LABELS ON FOOD. Many sugars are hidden.

BUY FRESH FRUIT. When selecting canned or frozen, choose those that are not in heavy syrup.

TRY TO DEVELOP A HABIT OF LESS SUGAR on cereals, in coffee or in tea.

SUBSTITUTE FOODS WITH LESS SUGAR FOR THOSE WITH HIGH SUGAR. For example, try fresh fruit as a snack instead of candy, or drink water or juice instead of soft drinks or punch.

AVOID TOO MUCH SODIUM

It is true that sodium is a mineral that is needed in the body, but most Americans consume too much sodium. High blood pressure is found in one out of four Americans. With it can come the risk of heart attack, stroke and kidney disease, and sodium may affect high blood pressure.

Sodium can come from the salt shaker - or the salt you freely add to foods when eating or cooking. However, a large proportion of sodium comes from hidden sources, like processed foods, commercially prepared foods, condiments, cheese, cold cuts and other foods. Remember, the fact that a food does not taste salty is not the key to the sodium amount — read the label instead.

It may be reassuring to know that you were not born with a preference for salt — you learned it. Perhaps, gradually reducing the amount of salt you eat will help to reduce the desire you have for it.

Other tips to reducing sodium include:

SELECT FRESH VEGETABLES INSTEAD OF CANNED.

EXPERIMENT WITH SPICES AND HERBS AS SEASONING INSTEAD OF SALT. Remember that garlic salt or seasoned salt still contain a lot of salt. Select garlic powder, onion powder or herbs.

DO NOT SALT THE WATER when cooking pasta or rice.

MAKE YOUR OWN SALAD DRESSINGS and store in the refrigerator.

United States Department of Agriculture, Human Nutrition Information Service, *Nutrition and Your Health, Dietary Guidelines for Americans*, Home and Garden Bulletin Numbers 232-1, 232-2, 232-3, 232-4, 232-5, 232-6 Washington DC, U.S. Dept. of Agriculture, April 1986.

ENTERTAINING MADE EASY

Nearly everyone is occasionally the host or hostess of an event. Whether it is a family dinner, children's party, or elegant reception, it need not be a time to panic. It is fun and easy to entertain if you plan.

Planning is the key to any successful event. Thinking through your ideas early and writing them all down frees your mind to carry out the tasks and to enjoy the event. Another added benefit of planning is that time and money management will result. You can spread your time and money expense out over a period of time, and you can prioritize so that you do and buy the most important things first.

Where to start planning? Contrary to popular belief, it is NOT with the food. The menu should come much later. Look at these steps.

1. EVALUATION. Evaluate you and what you really want. Consider when the party will be. What space is available? What is your budget?

Part of the evaluation is knowing the reason for giving the party. Sometimes, it is set — like the family's Thanksgiving Dinner or your daughter's birthday. Others center around specific happenings like a bridal shower, anniversary, or new home. Perhaps it is truly wanting to entertain friends.

Decide early if you are giving the event alone or if you need help. Must you reserve a place, rent tables, hire a caterer, arrange help or engage musicians? If so, determine these contracts before going any further.

2. SET THE THEME. Be creative, but remember your evaluation and the reason for the party. The theme is important because the entire event will be based on it, including food, music, decorations, and guest list.

It may be helpful to think of a couple different themes and compare them to your space requirement, budget and other known factors. Then you will be able to choose the one that really fits you and your guests best.

3. INVITATION LIST. Consider the invitation list carefully. There is no need for each one invited to be exactly alike, but they should mix well. Remember, it often shows if you invite someone only because you feel obligated.

4. MENU. What foods go with the theme? Will it be refreshments or a dinner? Will the meal be a sit-down affair or a buffet? What will the budget allow? Again consider your space, the type of service, your dishes and seating. A buffet is easy to serve, but if seating is limited, you may have to restrict the menu to finger foods.

Whatever the food is, it should be simple, attractively served and there should be plenty of it. Think of what foods can be done in advance, and what must be done the day of the party. Generally, the best party menus are ones in which very little must be prepared at the last minute.

5. MAIL INVITATIONS. Invitations should be sent (or guests called) about 2 weeks before the party or up to 1 month before for weddings or other major events. Be sure and include the date, time for the party to begin and end, place, and your own name, address and phone number. An R.S.V.P. (with a phone number noted) will help remind people to call and let you know if they are coming.

Be sure the invitation is clear and complete. For example, are children invited? Is Bob to come alone or bring a guest? Be sure and specify if a special event, like showing slides, or going out dancing is planned.

6. MAKE LISTS. Keep a detailed list of all that is needed. What can be done in advance and what must be done the day of the party?

7. DECORATIONS AND ARRANGEMENTS. What can be done to make it festive? What decorations will carry out the theme the best? Remember to plan serving bowls, napkins, garnishes and centerpieces as part of the decorations.

Think of your guests in all arrangements. It is usually best to clear away the rare and breakable. Clear off tables and provide coasters so guests can set drinks. Where will the pet stay? Are there fresh towels, soaps, and ashtrays. Is there plenty of ice?

8. ENJOY. The best parties are those that are given for fun and relaxation. The comfort of the guests is considered and all is done in a true spirit of friendship. Planning helps to make it possible and will add to the fun.

THE BEST USE OF YOUR FREEZER MAY MAKE MEALTIME EASIER

Is your freezer a mystery? Is it an empty, dark cave, filled with the unknown, or is it so full you can't see what is there?

Whatever its state, the fact that you have one can mean a real difference in meal planning. If you are interested in convenience, quality, and food variety, the freezer may hold the key.

These tips will help you use your freezer correctly.

FREEZE AT THE PEAK OF FRESHNESS. If you have a garden, this means freezing vegetables very quickly after picking. If it is your casserole, or the appetizers for next week's party, freeze it soon after preparing. Remember, the freezer will preserve food — not refresh it.

FREEZE FOOD QUICKLY. Quick freezing means that ice crystals are smaller and flavor and texture will be the best. Slower freezing means larger ice crystals and even more opportunity to reduce flavor and texture. Chill the food first in the refrigerator. Then, place the food to be frozen right on the shelf.

WRAP CAREFULLY. Wrapping must be moisture-proof and air-proof to prevent drying or freezer burn. The freezer is not a cold, still world; rather it is a constant motion of air currents and food must be protected. Select freezer wrap, heavy duty aluminum foil or specially marked plastic wrap. Many plastics (like store wraps or sandwich bags) are not moisture or air-proof.

KEEP THE FREEZER AT ZERO. Check this with a thermometer, not the hardness of food. It is possible for the food to "feel hard" but not be solidly frozen. If the food is not solidly frozen, the quality will decline.

FREEZE FOOD ONCE. Thawing food, then refreezing may destroy moisture, flavor, texture and nutrition.

LABEL THE FOOD. Contrary to what you might think, you will not remember what that funny shaped package is. Include the contents, and the date. If you note the cooking or heating instructions right on the label, others will know how to heat it.

KEEP FREEZER FULL. A freezer kept 75%-85% full will operate most efficiently.

USE THE FOOD - don't just save it. Plan to restock at least twice a year for optimum food flavor.

FOLLOW THE RULE OF FIRST IN - FIRST OUT. Rotate the food and use the oldest items first.

THAW FOOD PROPERLY - if at all. Some foods need no thawing before cooking. If thawing is required, thaw it slowly in the refrigerator or in a water-proof container in cold water.

BUY FROZEN FOOD WISELY. Be sure that the packages are solidly frozen and not heavily frosted. If it is frosted or misshapen, you will know that thawing has occurred and some quality was lost.

REFREEZE CAREFULLY. Refreezing may not cause a health hazard if the food is cold and some ice crystals remain. Discard any food that has an off odor or has an off color. If in doubt, do not refreeze. Do not refreeze ice cream, fish, shell fish or prepared dishes. Remember, quality will have deteriorated when any food is refrozen.

SOME FOODS ARE BEST NOT FROZEN — or, will change somewhat. For example, potatoes may become mushy. Fried foods may become soggy and stale. Lettuce and greens wilt. Milk or cheese sauce may curdle.

HOW LONG CAN FOOD STAY FROZEN? This is a general idea, based on optimum quality and flavor for foods held at 0° F.

Ice Cream	1 month
Fruits, Vegetables	Up to 1 year
Butter or Margarine	1 month
Ground Beef	2-3 months
Pork	4-6 months
Beef steak, Roast	Up to 1 year
Cooked meat, Poultry	1-6 months
Turkey	6-8 months
Lean Fish	6-9 months
Shell Fish	Up to 4 months
Baked Cakes	3-4 months
Baked Pies	1-2 months

Appliances can make many cooking tasks easier, faster and definitely more fun. Some, like toasters, coffee makers, or can openers are basic and are used often. Others are not as commonly used. This guide will give you some tips on operating some common appliances.

Remember, an appliance that is conveniently stored and easy to clean is used more often. Always remember to follow instructions and use appliances safely.

BLENDERS — These products are especially well suited for blending drinks and some will pulverize ice into frozen drinks. They are also excellent for blending salad dressing or pureeing a sauce.

To chop vegetables, the food must be covered with water. Drain vegetables before using.

When blending hot liquids, follow manufacturer's directions carefully. Many recommend removing the center cup from the cover first.

Do not over-blend. Blenders work quickly and chopped food will soon be pureed.

DEEP FRYERS — If you like to deep fry often, a deep fryer will make it easier since the temperature of the oil can be set for a specific food.

Remember not to overheat the oil. Set the temperature dial according to the recipe. If oil smokes, lower temperature immediately.

Use a good quality vegetable oil for deep frying. Do not use lard or butter.

ELECTRIC SKILLETS OR GRIDDLES — These may provide just the extra cooking space you need since they are so versatile. A griddle is perfect for pancakes, eggs, or sandwiches. An electric skillet can almost double as a griddle, but also will let you stir-fry, simmer, deep fry or do other cooking tasks.

FOOD PROCESSORS — These appliances now come in sizes that process from less than 1 cup up to 10 or more cups. Most were originally designed to quickly chop vegetables, and will conveniently chop, slice or shred cheese, nuts, vegetables, fruits and some meats. They make quick work of making baby food and spreads, and handle the preparation steps for many dishes. Larger, more powerful units will also make pie crust, quick breads, or even knead bread dough.

Never try to operate them without the cover. Blades are very sharp so handle with care.

Slice iceburg lettuce and it will be shredded perfectly for tacos.

Have cheese well chilled. Be sure fruit is free from seeds or pits.

Generally, they will not blend drinks or chop ice.

ICE CREAM FREEZERS — A renewed interest in ice cream has made the ice cream freezer a popular appliance to own. Models include the electric or manual version, as well as several newer types that use table salt or a coolant that does not require ice or salt.

Follow the manufacturer's recommendation in regard to type and volume of salt or ice to use. Ice cream that is frozen too quickly or too slowly may not have the creamy texture you want.

SLICERS — They are perfect for slicing a ham once a year, but they also make quick work of slicing roasts, cheese, pound cakes, quick breads or French breads. Slice refrigerator cookies for pretty trays. Slice lemons or oranges thinly to use as a garnish on a drink.

SLOW COOKERS — Slow cookers are designed to simmer food slowly. Cooking time for meat dishes is generally 8-12 hours. They are famous for cooking soups, stews or sauces but are also excellent for cooking less tender cuts of meat, casseroles and other dishes.

WAFFLE IRONS — While these are an old stand-by, you may now select standard waffle irons or those that are also griddles. The waffle irons are available as standard waffles or the deep, crisp Belgian waffle. Some will also make pizzelles, the thin Italian cookies.

WOKS — These appliances came from China and were designed for stir-frying, or cooking food quickly over high heat, while stirring rapidly. The efficient shape is also excellent for deep frying or steaming.

GIFTS FROM THE KITCHEN

The kitchen is generally used for preparing nourishing family meals. But more and more, the kitchen is becoming an art and craft studio or workshop for gifts.

Home spun items, homemade foods and other "kitchen-crafts" are really popular today. Perhaps there is no gift more desired than something made "especially for you" from the kitchen.

WHAT FOODS MAKE PERFECT GIFTS?

Any food item that you make especially well, is unique, or represents your cultural background is a wonderful gift.

Some ideas include:

Bread	Rolls	Muffins
Cakes	Cookies	Pies
Jams	Jelly	Candy
Flavored vinegars	Soup mix	Drink mixes
Relish	Pickles	Syrup
A favorite seasoning blend	Flavored nuts	

MAKE IT LOOK FESTIVE

Food will look extra festive and special if attractively presented. Try the stenciling idea, which follows, or look to pretty boxes, baskets, tins or other containers to give a special look.

Sometimes the container is really a part of the gift and will serve double duty. A set of glasses or mugs could each hold a different relish, jam or jelly. One coffee mug filled with candy, cookies, or nuts, and tied with ribbon might make the perfect gift for a child to give to the teacher. Fill a decorative cannister with a soup mix, and tie a soup ladle in with the bow. Fill a salad dressing cruet with an herb-flavored vinegar.

The wrap itself might also be functional as well as pretty. For example, a kitchen towel might wrap a bread, or napkins might wrap the jars filled with tea mix.

SPECIAL INSTRUCTIONS AND GIFT CARDS

Always tell the person how to serve the gift and include special information about storing. For example, specify if jam is to be refrigerated or frozen or note if the torte is filled with cream or cream cheese and must be refrigerated.

For a special touch, write the history of the dish, some serving ideas, how to store it and even the recipe on a decorative card and tie it to the package.

SOME GIFTS DO NOT REQUIRE COOKING

Gifts from the kitchen do not have to be the finished food. Try tying the ingredients for your favorite dish and the recipe together in a decorative basket. Or assemble some special ingredients for a certain type of cooking together on a tray or cutting board.

STENCILED OR PAINTED FOOD

Stencil or paint food to give a special look that is perfect for any holiday or party. It is also fun to personalize a food when giving it to a friend.

To make an edible paint, lightly beat together egg yolks. Blend in food coloring until the desired color is reached. Apply using a new, clean brush.

If desired, find a pattern or use a clean, new art stencil. Children's coloring books are also good sources of large pictures that can be traced.

Yeast bread and double crust pies are perfect for stenciling. Note these tips:

Bread — Yeast breads have a smooth crust that is easily painted. Paint or stencil after bread has baked and cooled.

Pie — Double-crust fruit pies are pretty stenciled with a holiday design or pictures of the fruit inside. Paint the crust after positioning on the pie, but before baking.

ADAPTING YOUR FAVORITE RECIPES TO THE MICROWAVE OVEN

Many of the family's favorite recipes came along before the microwave oven. However, just because your recipe is written for conventional cooking methods, there is no reason why you can't adapt some of them to this faster cooking method.

FIND A SIMILAR RECIPE IN YOUR MICROWAVE COOKBOOK AND USE IT AS A GUIDE. If it is a meat item, find a recipe that has a similar amount of the same kind of meat as your own recipe. The same is true of vegetables. Also, note the amount of liquid used and try to find a recipe with a similar amount. The similar recipe will help you know what size dish to use, what power setting to use, and what the cooking time might be.

KNOW WHICH FOODS ARE NOT REALLY SUITED TO THE MICROWAVE OVEN. Among them are crisp pastries, fried foods, breaded foods, and hard-cooked eggs in the shell. Also remember that some foods take longer to cook or just don't cook as easily in the microwave oven. For example, pasta may require the same time in the microwave oven as on the stove. If you cannot find a similar recipe in your microwave book, realize that there might be a reason it was not recommended.

TIMING IS BASED ON THE AMOUNT OF FOOD, THE AMOUNT OF LIQUID, THE STARTING TEMPERATURE AND YOUR TYPE OF MICROWAVE OVEN. Start with what you might think is a minimum time, then increase cooking time as necessary to achieve the desired doneness. It is helpful if you have made the dish before and know what the food looks like when done.

COOKING TIME WILL BE ABOUT ¼ TO ½ THE TIME USED IN CONVENTIONAL COOKING. Of course, this will vary with the points noted above. Foods that need to tenderize, like a beef chuck roast, will require more cooking time to obtain the desired tenderness, even in the microwave oven.

USE A MICROWAVE-SAFE CONTAINER. Be sure and allow adequate space for any boiling.

REDUCE LIQUIDS. Generally, dishes will require slightly less liquid than the conventional recipe did since there will be less evaporation. The exception is if rice or pasta is used as they will absorb moisture. In general, start with a minimum amount and add more during cooking if needed.

CHANGE THE SIZE OF THE PIECES OF FOOD. Small pieces of food, cut in uniform size, will microwave faster and more evenly. This may be especially true in casseroles or stews.

STIR OR REARRANGE FOOD. Remember to stir, rearrange food, or rotate the dish to achieve even cooking.

EASY ON THE SEASONINGS. Use less salt and adjust the seasonings after cooking.

APPETIZERS ARE PERFECT FOR THE MICROWAVE. Dips can be heated as long as the dish is safe for microwave cooking. Arrange appetizers on a serving plate and microwave until warm.

MOST BREADS, CAKES AND PIES ARE NOT SUITED FOR MICROWAVE COOKING. It is generally difficult to adapt these recipes to the microwave. Therefore it is best to use recipes specially developed for the microwave oven. Keep those favorites for when you have time to bake in the conventional oven.

USE A LOWER POWER SETTING WHEN COOKING EGG OR CHEESE DISHES IN THE MICROWAVE. Overcooking will toughen them.

FISH DISHES ARE PERFECT FOR ADAPTING TO THE MICROWAVE since they cook quickly. Use high power and watch cooking progress carefully to avoid overcooking.

NEVER TRY TO ADAPT YOUR CANNING RECIPES TO THE MICROWAVE OVEN.

GROUND BEEF DISHES GENERALLY WORK WELL IN THE MICROWAVE OVEN.

REDUCE THE BUTTER AND OIL. More butter or oil are used conventionally to prevent sticking. In the microwave, use just a little if you want the flavor.

FOREIGN FOODS ADD INTEREST TO MEALS

Many foods from around the world seem mysterious and intriguing since some people are not familiar with them. Others seem so common they don't appear foreign anymore. No matter, they are all wonderful and add new excitement to meals. The most popular foreign cuisines in the United States today are Mexican, Italian, and Chinese. This summary will introduce you to them and spark some ideas on how you might include their flavors in your everyday meals.

MEXICAN — This old and wonderful cuisine goes far beyond the tacos that many people are familiar with. Not every dish is hot and spicy. Tortillas, while popular and often served, are not the only food. There is an interesting mix of meat, fish, and seafood, served with rice or beans, and delicately seasoned with tomatoes, peppers, chilies, and seasonings such as coriander or cumin.

The dishes can easily be served as an entire feast or combined with your own favorites to add interest to a meal. Many Mexican snacks or appetizers are flavorful and would make wonderful additions to any appetizer trays. A Flan, or caramel custard, is the perfect dessert for any meal — light, sweet and refreshing. A dish that might enliven any brunch is scrambled eggs flavored with salsa, chorizo sausage or zucchini. Any gourmet will enjoy the flavor of Arroz con Pollo (Chicken with Rice).

Mexican flavors are fun to capture in your quick, everyday meals. Bottled salsa will make an excellent appetizer dip or baste for chicken as it bakes. Everyday baked beans will taste new if garbanzo beans and Mexican chorizo sausage are added.

ITALIAN — The Italian cuisine has offered us so much. We already love the spaghetti, pizza and lasagna. Many now love pasta in all forms — fresh or dried, in various shapes, various flavors and with sauces other than the typical tomato-based.

Italy has two distinct regions and therefore two distinct cooking styles. The Southern region gives us the pasta like spaghetti or macaroni that is made without eggs. The sauces are robust and are often made of tomatoes. Olive oil, artichokes, eggplant, pepper and garlic are common.

The Northern region has given us the flat pasta, like fettuccine, that is made with eggs. Butter and cream are popular. Rice is often served instead of pasta.

Together these regions give us a wonderful and varied cuisine. In addition to the pasta, the foods of Italy include seafood, veal, roasted meats, and wonderful sausages and hams. Cakes and pastries are delicious and rich.

Again, quick additions to your own meals might be a version of antipasto such as an appetizer like prosciutto ham wrapped around wedges of cantaloupe, or try mushrooms marinated in olive oil, and seasoned with garlic and oregano. A warm minestrone soup, a tomato-vegetable soup that contains zucchini and dry beans, will definitely take the chill off a cold evening.

CHINESE — The Chinese have given us a wonderful, old, cooking style that is new, fresh, and innovative. Their best known cooking style is the art of stir-frying.

There are five distinct regions of China and each offers a slightly different cooking style and seasoning. The Cantonese is probably the best known here.

Rice is definitely a staple of China. However, many dishes incorporate noodles. Vegetables, with a crisp texture, are of critical importance. Meat, fish, and poultry are also included.

One interesting aspect of the Chinese food culture is the beauty of the food. Colors are pure and eye appeal is almost as critical as flavor.

Fried rice, or frying rice with eggs and bits of ham, is a quick evening meal. The art of stir-frying can be borrowed and nearly any vegetable combination you happen to have in the refrigerator can be quickly made into a beautiful, tasty dish. Egg rolls or a sweet and sour sauce on shrimp are perfect appetizers for any meal. In addition, the current dietary trends, recommending less meat and more vegetables and starch, are very flavorful if prepared in the Chinese fashion.

ATTRACTIVE FOOD IS FUN AND EASY

How something looks really affects your enjoyment of it. You know that appearances can work against food -- like wilted lettuce or an off-color sauce. So too, the appearance can really enhance food. It can make a plain meal into a festive, special one. It will entice the picky eater to eat. It tells your family you are really glad to share dinner with them.

Appearance is a combined effort of color, texture, and shape. Think not only of the food itself, but also of the linens and dishes that will be used with the meal.

Gone are the days when we could only use white china and linen. Today's table is set with bright colored plastics on vinyl cloths. Or it is pastel stoneware on home-style mats. Colors once never used with food, like purple, or black, are now fine. We can even mix or match china, stoneware and baskets. This really means your creativity can soar. And the beautiful dishes and cloths need more than that old wilted sprig of parsley as a garnish.

Look at some new serving and garnishing ideas that will highlight your cooking, without taking up too much time.

SET THE MOOD. Establish a feeling or select the theme of the meal. Is it formal or informal? What kind of meal is it? What season of the year is it? This will help your creative thoughts plus give you ideas for linens to use, for centerpieces or other decorations, as well as help you select the food itself and how to serve it.

LOOK AT COLOR. Make sure there is a wide variety and that they go together. Most food colors "go together" so it is simply a matter of offering foods that have lots of different colors, then match the colors of the napkins, cloths or garnishes to the colors of the food. Offer pleasing contrasts and accents that make the food stand out and look its best.

LOOK AT STYLE. Some foods and events just naturally call for a certain style of presentation. Holidays are a perfect example.

Halloween seems to be an informal time, while Valentine's Day may fit any style but the presentation could include silver or candlelight.

Tastefully done, you can mix old and new, or silver with less-formal pieces. But do so with caution and a critical eye.

TEXTURES SHOULD ADD VARIETY. Textures can be interesting and really add to your presentation. Interesting mats over cloths, various baskets and other accessories really add to the interest.

SERVING PIECES. Serving pieces can be as varied as your imagination will allow and this is a really easy way to liven up the table. Use a variety of shapes and sizes of containers. Can an old book be gracefully wrapped in a napkin and used to hold an appetizer plate up at a different height? Arrange finger food on a footed cake server. Would old, antique glasses show off parfaits?

FOOD CONTAINERS. Look to food itself for the container. Hollow out a pumpkin and use it to serve a stew or a punch. Hollow out a green or red pepper to hold a dip. Remove the heart of a head of red cabbage and fill with slaw. Serve fruit salad from a melon or cantaloupe boat. Use your imagination, and the season of the year. Just be sure that the food used as a container is fresh, clean and well chilled.

MAKE ALL FOOD LOOK ATTRACTIVE. When preparing any food, look for methods to make the food look extra nice. Make it a habit to look at the food and see if there is a way to add a little color interest -- and see how fast the flavor interest climbs too. These ideas are easy and quick and will turn any good cook into that extraordinary cook.

A quick sprinkle of paprika, herbs, bread crumbs or slivered almonds will liven up a plain casserole.

Leave the peel on fruits if possible to add extra color.

Slice celery or carrots into pieces large enough that they can be identified and can add color to the rest of the dish.

Slice some foods straight across, while others at a diagonal.

Sprinkle toasted coconut over a cake or fruit salad.

x

Drizzle chocolate over a cake frosted with a white frosting.

Sprinkle croutons and shredded cheese over cups of soup. Thinly slice a lemon, orange, zucchini, tomato or other food that matches the flavor of the soup and float the pieces in the bowl.

Always toss sliced bananas or chopped apples into lemon juice to prevent darkening.

GARNISHES

CHOCOLATE LEAVES. The leaves are beautiful on a cake, or on top of the whipped cream on a chocolate cream pie.

Wash and dry fresh mint leaves. Melt semi-sweet chocolate morsels over hot, not boiling water. Let chocolate cool but not harden. Using a new, clean paint brush, paint chocolate on back (dull-side) of leaves. Place, chocolate side up, on plate covered with wax paper. Freeze about 10 minutes or until firm. Carefully peel off chocolate, starting at stem end. Keep chocolate leaves chilled until ready to serve.

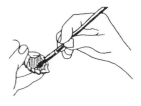

LEMON SPIRALS. Lemon spirals are one of the easiest and most versatile garnishes known. Use them on cakes, lemon meringue pie, nestled in parsley on a lemon-pasta dish, or on poultry or fish.

Select firm, deep yellow lemons. Do not peel. Slice full, thin, slices across center of fruit. On each slice, cut through peel and up just to center of the slice. Twist one half forward and one half backward.

Orange or lime spirals can be made in the same way.

FRUIT CUPS. Use fruit as a cup to hold colorful food accents.

Cut a scalloped pattern around an orange about ⅓ down. Discard top. Cut away fruit pulp from top. Fill with whole-berry cranberry sauce and place next to turkey or ham.

Cut a grapefruit in the same fashion and top with cherries for a breakfast or brunch garnish.

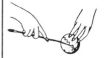

VEGETABLE CUPS. Thin slices of summer vegetables really dress up meat dishes when filled with relish.

Slice a zucchini, yellow squash or cucumber in slices 1-inch thick. Carefully spoon out the pulp, leaving the peel in an attractive ring. Fill with relish.

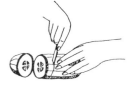

TOMATO ROSE. This elegant garnish is very popular today in gourmet restaurants, and really is easier than it looks.

With a very sharp knife, thinly peel a tomato in one, continuous strip, about ¾ inch wide. Gently, rewind the peel into a coil, with each coil fanning out a little to resemble a rose. Place on a bed of mint or basil leaves.

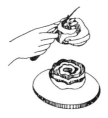

Saving Money

Being a wise shopper — one that knows value and how to save money — is easy to learn.

Remember that each family is unique. What you buy and how much you spend on food will depend on the number of people in your family, their ages, their specific health requirements, and of course, their personal flavor preferences.

No matter what the family — there are ideas that will help and tips that you can follow to stretch food dollars. Contrary to popular opinion, these ideas do not take a lot of time — saving time and money do not have to be totally opposite concepts.

PLAN — Plan the meals (which saves time too) and make a list of what you need. Avoid impulse buying.

USE COUPONS WHEN APPROPRIATE. Organize them and use them for the items you really need. Discard ones for products you really don't want or are for items your family really wouldn't use anyway.

STUDY THE ADVERTISEMENTS BEFORE SHOPPING. Check what is on sale and what is in season. See if you can plan your meals to take advantage of these money-saving offers.

EAT BEFORE SHOPPING. If you are hungry you will spend more money and be tempted to buy more.

SHOP ALONE. Children asking for treats and extras can add up to excess spending.

CHECK THE UNIT PRICE LABEL. Buy the cheapest unit price if it fits your use and your needs. For example, larger boxes may be the cheapest by unit price, but if you cannot use the entire item before spoiling, it won't be a good buy.

DON'T BE FOOLED BY FANCY PACKAGING. Check the real size in volume or weight and buy what you need. Sometimes boxes that look larger really hold less. Also, don't buy a product for the fancy container — buy for the item and quality inside.

CHECK STORE BRANDS. You probably will save by not paying for national advertising.

BUY THE CHEAPEST FORM OF THE PRODUCT THAT WILL SERVE YOUR NEEDS. For example, mushroom pieces and stems may work fine in a casserole, but sliced or even whole mushrooms might be needed for a company salad even though they cost a little more.

FRESH ITEMS, OR THOSE WITH THE LEAST PROCESSING, ARE GENERALLY THE CHEAPEST. Fresh produce is probably the cheapest if it is in season. Do check carefully as there are exceptions. For example, frozen orange juice is almost always cheaper than fresh.

TRY TO SHOP ONLY ONCE A WEEK. Staying out of the store is one of the best ways to avoid impulse buying.

LOOK FOR THE FRESHEST MEAT AND PRODUCE. Buy carefully if "marked down for quick sale." It is not a savings if you can't use it before it spoils.

CHECK ITEMS STACKED IN THE CENTER OF THE AISLE CAREFULLY. Is it really a special? Is the price really lowered? Can you really use it?

RESIST BUYING PRODUCTS YOU HAVE TASTED OR HAVE TALKED WITH A DEMONSTRATOR ABOUT. First, consider, will it fit into my menu plans for the week? Will my family really like it? Will the price fit into my budget?

A CLOSER LOOK AT CONVENIENCE PRODUCTS

Perhaps nothing in the grocery store offers more choices than the extensive line of convenience foods sold today. Convenience foods need careful evaluation in terms of the price. Often the price of packaged, convenience foods is higher than the cost of basic ingredients, but only you can make the best choice. What should you consider?

Realize that you are trading time for money.

Are you wanting to buy the cooking skill that you do not have?

Are each of the basic ingredients ones that you will use up or will the extra be wasted?

Is the dish really that difficult or take that much time to prepare?

SEASONING KNOW-HOW

More and more, you are told to use herbs or spices instead of salt, sugar, or fats.

They really do add flavor to the food and they are simple to use.

Is it an herb or a spice? Actually the word doesn't make much difference since both add wonderful flavor. The difference is that spices come from the roots, buds, flowers, fruits, bark or seeds, while herbs come from the leaves of plants.

Herbs come fresh or dried, in whole leaf, seed or ground form. Spices are available whole or ground.

Herbs and spices should be carefully stored as they will become stale or lose their flavor easily. Store them tightly covered, in a cool, dry place, away from the range. The flavor of herbs naturally weaken with age so buy small bottles and replace them often.

Dry herbs are more concentrated than fresh. If substituting fresh herbs for dried herbs, use 2 to 3 times more fresh herbs than dried.

Whole leaf herbs and whole spices will hold their flavor better during long cooking. If tied in cheesecloth, they are easy to remove before serving. Add ground herbs during the last 5-10 minutes of cooking. Ground spices give an almost instant flavor and are best for baking, or quick-cooking food.

Many herbs and seasonings are now available in blends, salts, or powders. A blend is simply a combination of herbs, spices and perhaps other seasonings like salt or sugar. Read the label carefully. Salts are combinations of an herb or spice and salt. Powder is the ground form of the seasoning.

COMMON SEASONINGS AND THEIR USE

ALLSPICE — Use in pickling, on baked ham, in baking cakes, cookies, in tomato sauce or soup.

BASIL — Use in soups, stews, sauces. Also good on eggs or pasta.

BAY — Use in soups, stews, in tomato dishes and in pickles.

CARAWAY — Popular in baking breads, cakes, or cookies. Use also on cabbage or beets.

CHIVES —Excellent on eggs, salads, or potatoes.

CINNAMON — Excellent on baked fruit, in fruit butter, on hot cereal or in baking cakes, cookies, pies, or breads.

CLOVES — Use in fruit dishes, on ham or pork, in baking cakes, cookies, pies, breads, or pastries or in pickling.

CORIANDER — Popular in pickling, in stuffing for poultry, on fresh pork or when making sausage.

DILL — Use in dips, on fish, in pickling or in making soups, stews, or sauces.

GINGER — Use in cakes, cookies, breads, on beef, in stews, on sweet potatoes or carrots.

MACE — Use in pickling or preserves, in cherry pie, in fruit cobblers, or in some sauces.

MARJORAM — Popular on chicken, in cheese or egg dishes, as a poultry seasoning or in salads.

MINT — Use fresh leaves in beverages. Use dried with fruit or in sauces.

NUTMEG — Use in sausages, on ham or pork, in baking cakes, cookies, or in egg-nog.

OREGANO — Use in tomato sauces, in beef stew, in pizza or in pasta dishes. It is an ingredient in chili powder.

PAPRIKA — Use it to season shell fish, salad dressings, and some beef dishes or stews. Its red color gives a finishing touch to many casseroles.

PARSLEY — A popular seasoning for many dishes, including sauces, stews, soups, egg dishes, or salads.

PEPPER — Available in red, black or white forms. It will provide zest for any dish, including salads, meats, soups, stews, casseroles, or fish, and is used in pickling.

SAGE — Use in sausage and in poultry dishes or stuffings.

THYME — Use in soups, stews, or sauces.

EQUIVALENTS • WEIGHTS • MEASURES • SUBSTITUTIONS

MEASURES • WEIGHTS

3 teaspoons	= 1 tablespoon
16 tablespoons	= 1 cup
8 tablespoons	= ½ cup
5⅓ tablespoons	= ⅓ cup
4 tablespoons	= ¼ cup
2 cups	= 1 pint
2 pints	= 1 quart
4 quarts	= 1 gallon
16 ounces	= 1 pound
8 ounces	= ½ pound
4 ounces	= ¼ pound

COMMON CAN SIZES

Picnic	10½-12 ounces
#300	14-16 ounces
#303	16-17 ounces
#2	20 ounces
#2½	27-29 ounces
#3	46 ounces
#10	6½ pounds

FOOD EQUIVALENTS

Butter	1 pound	= 2 cups
Cheese	4 ounces	= 1 cup
Chocolate morsels	6 ounces	= 1 cup
Cream	½ pint	= 1 cup liquid
		2 cups whipped
Crumbs		
graham	14 squares	= 1 cup
saltine	28 squares	= 1 cup
Flour	1 pound	= 3½ cups
Lemon	1 medium	= 2-3 tablespoons
Orange	1 medium	= ⅓ cup
Rice		
long-grain	1 cup	= 2-3 cups, cooked
pre-cooked	1 cup	= 2 cups cooked
Spaghetti		
cooked	7 ounces	= about 4 cups
Sugar		
Brown	1 pound	= 2¼ cups, packed
Confectioners	1 pound	= 3-4 cups, unsifted
Granulated	1 pound	= 3 cups

SUBSTITUTIONS

For:	Substitute:
1 tablespoon cornstarch	2 tablespoons flour
1 cup self-rising flour	1 cup flour + 1 tsp. baking powder + ½ tsp. salt
1 cup cake flour	1 cup minus 2 Tbsp. sifted all-purpose flour
1 ounce unsweetened chocolate	3 Tbsp. cocoa + 1 Tbsp. fat
1 cup buttermilk or sour milk	1 Tbsp. vinegar or lemon juice + milk to equal 1 cup
1 cup honey	1¼ cups sugar + ¼ cup liquid

SOLVING THE "NO-TIME DILEMMA"

Nearly everyone is busy and, at least occasionally, faces a dilemma over how to stretch time. There are some tips that really do help you to better utilize the time you have and make it seem like more.

FIRST STEPS TO SAVING TIME

Just like a doctor evaluates your health before prescribing treatment, you too must evaluate your time before making changes. Keep a log of your activities, noting what you were doing, the time of day and how long it took. Note whether the task was a priority, a routine task or did it have no purpose at all? Did you feel alert, energetic, neutral or sluggish?

Evaluate your log after a week. Did you really live out your priorities? When you were doing your hardest tasks, did you feel energetic or sluggish? Did you realize how long it took to do each job?

Now understand that you are the executive of your own time. You are in the position to make decisions. Can you allow more realistic time to each priority task? Can you rearrange tasks? Can others help with certain tasks?

Now that you have evaluated your use of time, you can make improvements.

MAKE LISTS. Free your mind for more important information. Begin with things to do today. Write down everything, then prioritize. Star the most important or put them at the top of your list.

PLAN THE NIGHT BEFORE. Set aside about 15 minutes each evening to plan the next day's activities.

DIVIDE LARGE PROJECTS INTO SMALL SEGMENTS that can be accomplished daily or at least weekly.

REALLY USE YOUR BEST TIME. Set aside your peak activity time for your most difficult project. Keep less demanding tasks for less productive times of day.

MAKE CHOICES. No one can really do it all.

PLAN REWARDS. Crossing off items on your list is very satisfying. So is extra time for a hobby or special event after completing a major project.

PLAN THE UNEXPECTED. Build in a margin in every plan. Do not become a strict sergeant or you'll defeat the purpose of your efforts, which was to make your life easier and more pleasant. Your life is not predictable; the unexpected will occur and accidents do happen. Your plan and organizational skills will free you from some of the stress and perhaps you can now enjoy life's surprises.

LESS TIME IN THE KITCHEN

Even if your hobby is cooking, there are times when you must minimize cooking time. Check these ideas.

PLAN YOUR MEALS AND PURCHASES. Planned meals are faster to fix, since you don't have to stop and stare at the pantry and think "what will it be tonight?" You will also avoid the problem of not having the right ingredients.

MINIMIZE SHOPPING. Since your meals are planned a shopping trip is easier and faster. Nothing eats up more time than stopping at the grocery store every day. Limit your shopping to once every week or even once every two weeks.

POST THE MEAL PLAN. Then, anyone home first can start the meal and the excuse of not knowing what to fix will be eliminated.

ORGANIZE YOUR SHELVES AND FREEZER. Keep them well stocked and know where items are. Keep some quick meals at your finger tips. A few minutes spent in organizing now will save lots of time in the future.

COOK IN LARGER BATCHES. Double or triple a recipe and freeze portions in heat-sealed boilable bags or microwave-safe cooking bags. Freeze family-size or individual-size servings. Cook extra meat and plan to use it in casseroles, soups, salads or sandwiches. A frozen casserole can easily bake while you are free to do other tasks. A well-stocked (and well-labeled) freezer will be a wonderful resource of quick-to-heat meals.

SIMPLIFY MEALS. Plan to use one-dish meals.

PACK LUNCHES THE NIGHT BE-
FORE AND REFRIGERATE. Many sandwiches can even be prepared for the whole
week and kept frozen.

TAILOR THE MEAL TO THE EVE-
NING. Realize that some evenings de-
mand a quick meal while sometimes the
best arrangement is for the meal to cook
"by-itself" in the oven or slow cooker while
you are busy with other things.

MINIMIZE CLEAN-UP WHEN POSSI-
BLE. Line roasting pans with aluminum
foil. Many casseroles can be cooked,
served and stored in the refrigerator in one
container.

MINCE ONION OR GREEN PEPPER
when you have a minute and freeze for use
in sauces, soups or stews later.

KEEP AND USE DRY MINCED
ONION. Also keep dry herbs, especially
those like parsley. Use about ½ of the dry
as you would fresh.

SOME FOODS ARE NATURALLY
QUICK COOKING. Included are eggs,
cheese, fish, and seafood. In these cases,
do not overcook.

USE PLASTIC FOOD BAGS TO SAVE
CLEAN-UP. Marinate meat in them. Fill
with seasoned bread crumbs, add chicken
pieces and shake to coat. Shake cookies in
a bag to coat with sugar.

SHREDDED CHEESE CAN BE FRO-
ZEN for use later.

OVERLAP RECIPE STEPS. Do all the
chopping, or measuring for a meal at one
time.

PREPARE BASIC MEATBALLS AND
FREEZE. Then heat and serve with a different sauce for exciting meals. Serve with
spaghetti sauce, a barbecue sauce, brown
gravy or sweet and sour sauce.

WHEN IS IT FASTER NOT TO MEA-
SURE? Many casseroles, soups, stews and
sauces will taste fine if you adjust the recipe
a little. Use a stalk of celery or the whole
onion instead of measuring exactly. However, measuring accurately when baking is
essential.

MAKE EXTRA WAFFLES AND
FREEZE. Pop into your toaster on busy
mornings.

KEEP INDIVIDUAL SERVINGS of
cake, muffins, rolls, coffee cake, biscuits,
or cookies frozen. They are ready to heat
for a quick breakfast or pack for lunch.

CLEAN WHILE COOKING. The five
minutes that a sauce simmers may be the
perfect time to clean out one drawer or un-
load the dishwasher.

MORE TIPS ABOUT THE HOUSE

HANDLE PAPER ONCE. Throw away
"junk mail" immediately or correctly file
those to keep.

MAKE IT A HABIT TO KEEP EVERY-
THING IN ITS PLACE. Looking for lost
tools, shoes, or whatever is aggravating,
and wastes time.

SET THE RIGHT PACE EACH DAY.
Set out clothes, books, bags, or whatever
the night before. Set the breakfast table. Do
all that you can to make your morning go
smoothly and start the day in an organized,
efficient and peaceful manner.

USE COLOR WHENEVER YOU CAN.
Color-code clothes for each child and provide a laundry basket the same color to
speed sorting. The "Red" drawer always
has Mom's red scissors, red pens, and
other red office supplies that stay by the
phone. The green file always has the
Christmas card and gift lists while the blue
notebook has the medical records.

KNOW THAT MANY JOBS EXPAND
TO FIT THE TIME AT HAND. Therefore,
limit the time. Set the timer and pick up all
you can before the time is up. Same way
with weeding the garden or whatever the
task is.

TRY TO BE MORE ALERT. Change the
order something is done. Make a game of a
task. Plan a new way to drive to work. Give
yourself a 5 minute stop at a favorite shop.

LIMIT PHONE CALLS. Set aside some
time and make them all at once. Use an an-
swering machine to answer calls during
your busy "productive time."